Planning for Survival

A Handbook for Hospital Trustees

Second Edition

Norman H. McMillan

American Hospital Publishing, Inc.,
a wholly owned subsidiary
of the American Hospital Association

The views expressed in this book are those of Norman H. McMillan.

Library of Congress Cataloging in Publication Data

McMillan, Norman H., 1925-
   Planning for survival.

1. Hospitals—Planning.   2. Hospitals—Trustees.
I.   Title. [DNLM: 1. Governing Board—handbooks.
2. Hospital Administration—United States—handbooks.
3. Hospital Planning—United States—handbooks.
WX 39 M478p]
RA971.M434 1984 362.1'1'068 84-24578
ISBN 0-939450-53-4

Catalog no. 127174

Beryl Dwight, Editor
Gretchen Messer, Production Coordinator
Marjorie E. Weissman, Manager, Book Editorial
Dorothy Saxner, Vice-President, Books

For Marge

Contents

Foreword

As a trustee of two hospitals and a rehabilitation center, Norman H. McMillan observed that business techniques for long-range planning are not routinely used by hospitals. Because he believes the process can and should be adopted by all hospitals and other health care institutions, he calls on hospital trustees, administrators, and medical staffs to accept the possibly unfamiliar, but successful, ways of planning he describes in this book.

In this, the second, edition, he describes such components of the current health care environment as prospective pricing, preferred provider organizations, and business coalitions and emphasizes the resulting increased need for improved strategic planning by today's health care institutions.

McMillan, who is widely known for his work as a hospital trustee over the past 25 years, is currently a consultant to the Task Force on Marketing and Referrals, University of Chicago Medical Center, and a member of the Council for the Division of the Biological Sciences and the Pritzker School of Medicine, University of Chicago. He is a former chairman of the board of trustees of St. Mary's Rehabilitation Center, Minneapolis, and a former member of the board of governors and chairman of the long-range planning committee of Methodist Hospital, Minneapolis. Prior to that, he was on the board of Methodist Hospital, Philadelphia. He has also taught a course in independent study for health care trustees at the Center for Health Services Research, School of Public Health, University of Minnesota.

Introduction

This book is about strategic planning for hospitals. It is a book for the concerned trustees, administrators, and physicians who observe that many hospitals are in crisis and that more will soon be on the endangered species list. It is a call for a new kind of planning effort, a better way to anticipate hospitals' problems, a better way to plan the future for those who need a way to set things in order.

What is described here is a process, a way to peel back the protective layers of tradition that make it tough to understand the real issues; a way to uncover and identify the sacred cows, which may be a problem at your hospital; and a way to drive deeper into the planning process to show you how to develop answers to the problems that now crowd the horizon.

Getting answers, getting action, getting your hospital to move in the best interests of all the people it serves is what this book is about. Think of it as a survival manual at a time when hospitals are very much threatened.

Three Basic Premises

Here are the three premises I start with; call them biases if you like.

Premise 1 is that diversity in the hospital system is valuable and should be preserved. The range now is wide:

- From small to huge
- From narrowly specialized hospitals to giant multipurpose medical centers
- From rural to urban
- From Catholic, Jewish, and Protestant to nonsectarian

1

- From hospitals that are mostly advanced first-aid stations to hospitals in the educational spectrum

Out of this diversity have come a lot of good ideas and new ways to help sick people feel better. Because good ideas and good treatment are not focused in just one part of the country, one big university, one kind of hospital, one program, or one plan, I am for preserving the system's diversity. I am against narrowing the choices, against the idea of a single kind of care, universally dispensed. The maximum good will be served, the maximum number of people will be helped, and patient costs will be lowest when diverse methods are allowed to serve the diverse needs of our society.

Premise 2 is that government agencies are poor planners. Their record is not impressive. Although I want to believe that government agencies know what they are doing, my experience says to look out, be careful. Alarms go off in my head each time I am involved with health planning agencies.

Trustees who have been around a few years should reflect on their hospital's past experiences with government agencies. Some hospitals are still trying to dig out of the shambles created by the government planners who encouraged the building of extended care centers 20 years ago. Such centers were the big idea then; they are today's big headache in many hospitals. In one where I was personally involved, construction was encouraged, and then the planners' attention shifted. Funds went to newer schemes, and a 250-bed extended care center was left high and dry, beached like a big whale. Only now, many years later, are its vital signs saying that it can get off the critical list.

Experiences like that create biases. They should make you cautious around government planners. Never forget you are the one who picks up the pieces when a government plan runs your hospital into trouble. It is *your* hospital, *your* balance sheet, *your* patients, *your* community when things go wrong. You are in charge of all screwups, morally and legally in charge. Never forget it.

Premise 3 is that hospitals have generally done an inadequate job of planning. They can, should, and *must* do better.

Having stated my cautious outlook on government planning, I must in fairness state that the legislators moved into a vacuum created by the hospitals. Hospitals failed to plan and wasted resources. They failed to think ahead and did not meet some real community needs. They failed to anticipate the future even in the most rudimentary ways and blew some big bucks. They failed in a lot of ways, and the public stood up and demanded that something be done. The hospitals invited legislation.

The result is just about a standoff, then. Hospitals have been inadequate as planners, and government planners have not demonstrated their superiority.

My urgent plea is that hospitals take charge of their own future. Not just meeting the mechanical requirements of government planning agencies, but really planning. And not just reacting to the recently formed coalitions of business organizations (who have a big stake in the high costs of medical care).

For years Congress has been saying it, and now employers looking at their health care costs are saying it: *"You* plan, *you* figure out where you are going; *you* do it, *or we will!"* And they are probably right. If hospitals cannot figure it all out, someone else has to.

If hospitals really try, if they give it their best shot, if they really begin to organize their future better (that is what planning is all about), they can recapture control of their own destiny and can do much to move the government in sensible directions. There is much to be hopeful about.

Summing Up

I have stated three premises:

- Diversity in the hospital system should be preserved as the source of ideas and progress. We shouldn't discard what we've got without clearly proven alternatives in sight.
- The government's record in health care planning is poor, and its plans must be viewed with great caution. The planning being done by the various business coalitions is untested.
- Hospitals' record is not noticeably better, and they now must hustle, do better, outthink the government planners, and fill the vacuum they themselves created.

The survival of your hospital as you know it today is at stake.

3

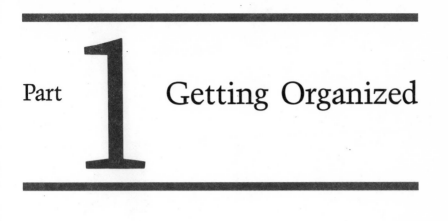

Part **1** Getting Organized

What Crisis?

You've seen the cartoon that says, "Show me a man who remains calm while all around are in a panic, and I'll show you a man who doesn't know what is going on." Something like that is going on in hospitals now. If you don't see big problems ahead of you, there is a high probability it is only because you are looking back at where your hospital has been, not feeling today's realities, not sensing the crisis ahead.

Item: Think about how the environment has changed over the past few years for all institutions: schools, businesses, churches, government, and *hospitals*. People are more suspicious, less trusting. More demanding, quicker to find fault, quicker to complain. More inclined to put your name in the paper. Faster on the draw, quicker to pull the trigger. It is a tougher environment for everyone to operate in. There are lots of signals that the terrain is unfriendly. Institutions of all kinds live in unfriendly times.

Item: Think about the unreasonableness of a society that demands the highest quality medical care and simultaneously acts shocked, surprised, and hostile when the rates are raised. When people are sick, they all want fancy equipment; high-powered, seldom-used gear; and teams of experienced medical specialists. And they want good food, instant service, and fancy rooms, too. But when they are well, it is a different story. Think about where it all leads and why the conflict.

Item: Think about all the government agencies that are looking into the high costs of health care and, in the process, have forced costs up by adding to the paper processing burden. Maybe one of the fastest rising costs of all is the cost of filling out all the forms for the various agencies looking into the high costs of health care.

Item: Think about your highly educated, knowledgeable friends, who ought to know better but who bellyache about the cost of a hospital

7

stay. The next time someone tells you your hospital charges more per day than the Waldorf Astoria, you might suggest that he check in there and call room service when he gets sick!

Item: Think about insurance plans that are running deficits. Think about government agencies, the biggest of all third-party payers, and the fact that they are now setting prices for your hospital's services regardless of your costs. Think about the emerging science of getting-paid, the result of government accounting practices. It is the newest medical specialty: how to fill out forms; how not to spend money, even when needed, because the government won't allow it. What does it mean, and where will it lead?

Item: Think about the fact that doctors and nurses can no longer make entries on the patient's medical chart as if it were solely for reference in future therapy or medical audit purposes. Think about the fact that the medical chart has been converted by the Medicare/Medicaid bureaucrats into an important tool for determining government reimbursement of patient care. This means doctors must be careful about what they write on the chart for fear some person in a distant city will declare that the government won't pay.

Item: Think about how your hospital would respond if the biggest employers in your town all got together, ganged up, and announced that, regardless of your costs, they were going to reduce the prices they would allow you to charge.

These things are happening now; they are not a prediction of things that could happen in 10 years. Now. Big change is under way, already programmed, being worked on. If you as a trustee are not involved, not aware, not studying, not participating in a task force, you are about to be a participant in a head-on collision.

Crisis just might be the most overworked word in the language today, and that is a pity, because crisis is what you've got on your hands. Hospitals are in crisis. They need leadership from their trustees as never before.

Crisis, the Perfect Moment for Planning

Let's face it: institutions do not change direction when things are going well. Businesses seldom change course when everything is going well and they have the luxury to do so in a neat, tidy way. Maybe it is the human condition; change is not generally the result of carefully laid plans made in times of tranquility, when there is leisure to be rational. In such times, management only *talks* about change. Governments react the same way, and hospitals are no better. They might even be worse, because they are perfectly programmed for stalemate. Many of them lack the clear-cut hierarchy of authority found in business that enables corrective action to be initiated when times get tough.

No, basic changes in direction do not come in good times. Change generally emerges from crisis. And that is exactly where hospitals are now. The crunch is here, and coping is no longer enough. In fact, it is one of the problems. Hospitals have muddled through so many problems for so long that it is hard for them to recognize that the crisis is real.

Although it is a scary time, it is also a time of great, probably unique, opportunity. This is it, the moment in history when planning pays off, the moment when the big chips all come out on the table, the precise time when you can get results because enough people can be made aware that the crisis is real. Not piles of paper, not pounds of plans, but action, movement, and results can be produced.

Your first problem, or the first stop on the road to survival, is to get your key decision makers aware of the crisis. You will find that a majority of the board and the medical staff cling tenaciously to the hope that "Everything is going to be all right. Everything will return to normal." Your first need is to create real understanding of the crisis your institution faces. Only when the alarm bells have been heard and their significance understood will there be enough adrenaline flowing to make the big decisions ahead. So you must begin with an educational effort, and it will be dry and tedious and hard, but essential. Here are some suggestions:

- Put together a seminar for your trustees that shows the statistical history of your hospital including all costs, income data, occupancy rates, and so forth. Now project the trends out 10 years. What do you see? (Most hospitals see disaster because costs have been increasing at a much faster rate than income.)
- Put together a meeting with the representatives of the biggest employers in your community. Ask them to present their data for the past 10 years on the cost of health care benefits to employees. Be sure to have your trustees and medical staff present so they can soak in these numbers. They will begin to understand the pressures better and to see the future with greater clarity.
- Put together a seminar on health planning legislation. Bring in the government planners so that the board of trustees and medical staff members can feel their impact. Plenty of them understand it intellectually, but few have it in their guts yet.
- Clip all of the articles on health care appearing in the past year in the *Wall Street Journal*. Read them, and sort them into two piles: negative and positive impact on your hospital. You will be pained by the lopsidedness of the piles. Then sort them again into two piles, according to whose ideas are being discussed: hospital-originated and government agency ideas. Again you will be pained. Sort them once more: cost issues and quality issues.

These are modest ideas, ways to get your associates to sense the crisis. Survival begins here; you need to know you are in trouble.

Predictable Statements You Will Be Too Wise to Believe

A key fact of life about planning in the hospital environment is that it is a political jungle. You must not be naive about it. Various departments of the medical staff battle for supremacy, for the rights to use certain equipment and to do certain procedures. They scrap for the hospital's investment dollars. Nursing management has jurisdictional disputes with almost everyone: the doctors, the pharmacy, the administration, among themselves; the hands-on nurses put down the supervisors and the teachers. A big front-office force deals with the flood of paper and forms needed to treat people, to collect bills, and, above all, to meet the requirements of the government agencies, the insurance companies, and "the Blues" so that the hospital can get paid. And for good measure, unions are now involved. It isn't easy to juggle these relationships.

Hospitals, it has been said many times, are labor, or people, intensive. This is true, but what *isn't* said is that hospitals are also ego intensive, the arena for the clash of some of the biggest egos around. There are a lot of individuals in the administration, the medical staff, the nursing staff, and even the board who are convinced that their training has equipped them uniquely to dictate answers to all management problems.

Hospitals, it has also been said, are the scene of life-and-death struggles. This, too, is true. They are places where everyone's emotions are wrenched and pounded all the time; and a lot of this emotion and conflict, this thunder and lightning, gets carried into the decision making. A hospital is a tough place to work in, a tough place to get consensus, a tough place to manage and maintain direction.

So it will be said to you about 15 minutes into your first discussion with other trustees that therefore the hospital cannot be planned. "This is not a business" is the opening put-down. "Hospitals are different; we must react to life-and-death emergencies." (That means hospitals must have a blank check.) "You cannot predict new medical developments, but you must be ready for whatever happens." That is the universal excuse for doing nothing—a kind of stalemate statement.

It will be said to you that the government is the source of most of the events that jar your hospital. "How can you predict what those fellows in Washington will do?" It is easy, as a matter of fact. Just listen to your radio and read your newspaper, and you can predict with certainty where government is headed with about three to five years' lead time. Many people in hospitals are looking for places to dump their responsibilities, and it is convenient to blame government.

It will be said with a faint smile through clenched teeth, "No one can predict what the medical breakthroughs will be in the next 10 years. Therefore we are wasting our time planning." This statement is appealing, but the grain of truth here is embedded in a wad of sticky thinking. For your purposes, as a planner, you can deal with uncertainty by building in flexibility.

It will be said in outrage, "You are dealing with human beings! You can't plan this place like a business and organize its future." Yes, hospitals are different, but the statement still assays out 90 percent pure baloney. The statement "We are different" is the universal cop-out for all business and institutional leaders who do not want to plan.

For sure, planning is not a perfected process, and you will hear that many times. Here is what planning really is:

- Thinking ahead
- Worrying about the future
- Learning and thinking about the enterprise, your hospital
- Anticipating problems, getting set for them
- Reading the environment
- Finding out what is wrong now so that you don't keep repeating mistakes
- Figuring out what is dividing your people, causing you to burn 10 times more energy than you should for the progress you make
- Accurately assessing your strengths and weaknesses, so that you know what you have to work with
- Figuring out what *might* be the alternatives—and picking one, not just drifting

- Setting a course and declaring it, getting everyone to support and rally around it
- Avoiding mistakes, not all mistakes, but a lot
- Getting a higher batting average, a higher ratio of good decisions to bad ones

So planning is not perfect, not mysterious. It is, quite simply, an organized way of applying common sense and judgment to your hospital's decision-making process. You are obligated, morally and legally, to do it. You don't really have a choice. You can plan for and anticipate the problems of your hospital, or you can sit back and react, waiting for others to control your destiny. So when they say, "We can't plan . . . ," press on, regardless. The option of not planning is not open to your hospital. You do it, others do it and impose their will on your hospital, or you go out of business.

Outside Influences

Maybe it is time to lay the cards face up about strategic planning.

There is a lot in the environment that is hostile to your hospital's future. And there is a lot out there that your hospital cannot control. But not knowing about it, or ignoring it, or acting as if it doesn't exist is no help. On the contrary, it guarantees a future full of unpleasant surprises.

A strong planning effort will not reduce the hostility in the environment a bit. Nor will an effective planning effort allow you to control all the situations the hospital will encounter. But a good strong planning effort will, absolutely, reduce the amount of negative surprise you deal with, and it will give you the advantage of time to create innovative responses.

Not bad. A good solid planning program at your hospital will give you the time you need to come up with better answers. And it is going to reduce the bad-news surprises you've been getting.

Some of the outside influences currently having an impact on your hospitals should be noted.

- *DRG.* This set of initials has been floating around in the jargon of hospitals for some time. It means *diagnosis-related group*, and it is part of the prospective pricing system that government now uses to pay hospitals for services to Medicare inpatients. Unlike the earlier system of cost-based reimbursement, prospective pricing assigns each Medicare patient to a DRG based on the nature of the illness, and each DRG carries a specific rate of payment.

   That sounds reasonable enough until you look at your own specific hospital. Maybe the payment established by prospective pricing will allow you to break even, maybe not. Maybe it will allow you to replace facilities as they wear out, maybe not. Maybe you can afford to treat your current mix of patients (or diagnosis-related groups), but maybe not.

The thing that you, as a trustee, need to know is that there is a big development affecting the cash flow of your hospital and you must be studying it so you can prepare the appropriate response.

Today it is DRGs. Tomorrow it may be something else. Viewed in the context of the long history of your hospital, it is only one more in a long stream of "hits." There will be more. And as a trustee concerned about the future of your hospital, not just the present, you should be on top of them, anticipating what comes next.

- *Business Coalitions.* Not all the pressure originates in Washington. These days, plenty of it starts with business people who are angry and frustrated about what they regard as out-of-control medical costs for employees. Those of us who are both hospital trustees and business executives find ourselves torn apart on this issue. As trustees, we see the threat to the well-being of the hospital; as business people, we are just as indignant as the next person at costs we cannot control.

Laying that aside, what we see here is a powerful new force to reckon with—it is the consortium of a group of major employers who get together in your town, on your doorstep, to do something about the high costs of medical care.

This is usually done with lots of publicity, full coverage from the newspapers, and if you play your cards wrong, you will get to see yourself in 90 seconds' worth of TV footage on the evening news—probably looking like a gouger, not the public-spirited trustee you thought you were.

Business coalitions are here and are probably going to become more important. You should understand their potential, their power, in your hospital's future.
- *PPO.* That's more hospital code, meaning *preferred provider organization*, which is still more code, obviously, and needs more translation. A preferred provider organization serves as a broker to work out a deal between a hospital and a business, or several businesses, or other parties, providing lower prices in exchange for a volume of business.

Some hospitals have gone into PPO arrangements, finding advantage. Others are resisting them fiercely. The point being made here, however, is a very simple one. This is a relatively new development that can influence your hospital's financial strength significantly. It is another outside influence you must measure, and decide what you want to do.

- *Doc-in-the-box*. Have you noticed everywhere you go lately there is a new presence – the storefront doctors' offices? Offices that are open all day, every day? Hours that match shopping hours, which is when most people are home from work? No appointments, just come on in whenever you need to see a doctor? Costs are $24 to $30 a visit, instead of a ton, like the hospital's emergency department? Doctors that call *you* the day after your visit to see how you feel?

  That's Doc-in-the-box, and it is a big development, obviously filling a void. It is wonderful to a lot of people.

  And it should be scary to a lot of hospitals. As many as 25 percent of the patient visits in some suburban Chicago locations are now occurring in these circumstances. That's great if your hospital is the referral center for the physicians working in these facilities. That's bad if the Doc-in-the-box around the corner from your hospital is sending referrals to another hospital.

These are examples of outside influences, the kind of phenomena that must be consciously observed and absorbed into your planning process. It is the job of the board to know about these things so it can develop the strategy of the hospital and keep the administration and medical staff challenged.

It is a big job. The list keeps changing. Several years ago it was the health planning act, Public Law 93-641, that scared the pants off the hospital industry. Now there are other influences. To those who thought hard about their strategy and kept a tight surveillance on the health care environment, the changes were not a shock, just another turn of the same wheel. To many others, the new developments have been startling and threatening.

The message is this. In a changing environment you will enhance the odds for survival of your hospital considerably just by insisting on a methodical, careful watchdogging of all that is going on around you.

Issue-Oriented Planning: Facing the Music

The trouble with most planning efforts is that they do not seek out the issues, face them, smack them on the nose, and get them resolved. Most planning efforts, instead, begin with solutions and then look for problems to solve. Most groups prefer to deal in answers. The principal fault of much government health care planning in the past, for example, is that it appears to have begun with bright ideas and then to have gone in search of a reason for being. The answers are more fun to play with. This is the act of creativity, like inventing; and everyone wants to do *that*.

Finding and facing issues is tough, slogging work, a lot of grunting, a lot of sweat, no fun; and no one wants to do *that*. But it is the essential A in the ABCs of strategic, or long-range, planning.

It is important to make clear that we are *not* talking about financial planning. That is a different animal; your hospital already does that. Your hospital makes certain assumptions and then forecasts costs and revenues for the year or years ahead. You will find, however, if you look carefully, that you simply have been pushing your trends ahead. If usage of the emergency department was up 17.5 percent last year and 17.6 this year, you will project the increase to be 17.7 percent for the next year.

Your financial planning should take into consideration events that will alter the hospital's finances. For instance:

- *Financial planning assumption 1.* The chief of the orthopedic service is 64½, has his house up for sale, and has just bought a home a thousand miles away in San Diego, near his grandchildren.

17

Therefore, you assume that the $500,000 a year in business he brings to your hospital won't be there next year, particularly since his young assistant has already declared his intent to join a prestigious group at another hospital. That is a financial planning assumption.

- *Financial planning assumption 2.* In recent years nurses' salaries have increased about 7 percent per year. But you've heard about union activity in neighboring hospitals, and according to the grapevine there are problems with your director of nurses. Your administrator has just reported a survey of other hospitals that shows your pay scales are about 6 percent under the average. You therefore assume a big jump in the nursing services expenditures next year, so you plug in a 15 percent increase. That, too, is a financial planning assumption.

These are examples of the kind of planning assumptions most hospitals work with—not too difficult to anticipate and figure about a year ahead.

But there are issues buried in those assumptions, such as:

- How did the doctor get to be 64½ without the hospital having planned a replacement strategy—a replacement that the community must have and that is of vital importance to the hospital's economics? How did that happen? *That* is an issue. If you don't come to grips with it, your hospital and the people it is intended to serve will get more blows just like that.
- How come the personnel practices have been allowed to get the hospital in a jam in so vital a sector of patient care as nursing? Why is it so late picking this intelligence off the grapevine? How did it get behind in paying the nurses? And *that* is an issue.

An issue, then, is more than a problem. It is an underlying cause of problems, the kind of thing that will just keep causing problems if it isn't fixed. And issue-oriented planning is different from financial planning. Think of an issue as a problem *generator:* resolve it or fix it, and you get rid of a *bunch* of problems.

Issues are all of the things that, if they could be fixed, you could say, "Our hospital does not have problems" and mean it. Most of all, issues are the things that cause the most divisiveness in your hospital, the things that prevent progress. Issues divide the hospital's key players.

Issues are hard to identify and incredibly hard to get discussed. If you think otherwise, go back to the example of the 64½-year-old orthopedic surgeon who is retiring—to the surprise of the hospital. Assume that the joint conference committee of the medical staff, board of trustees, and administration has met to discuss the situation. It is quite predictable that on the first go-around the following will take place:

- The administration will look to the medical staff for answers.
- The doctors will figure the administration goofed.
- The board will wonder in consternation how this event could have transpired, because for three years good old Doc Blank has been talking over the bridge table about moving to San Diego.
- With nothing having been settled, the committee members will agree at the end of the meeting that the problem will be investigated and another meeting will be scheduled. (Isn't that what you always do when faced with a problem?)

Now, with a little digging, some new information begins to emerge, and—surprise!—it is decided the information is too "delicate" and potentially inflammatory to discuss in an open meeting. It is also said that everyone knows this to be true, which would seem to indicate it has been discussed all over the place. What comes out is:

- The retiring orthopedist is a tyrant, and no one can work for him. Everyone in town knows it, but you.
- The facilities provided for the orthopedic department are outmoded, and some of the equipment that newly licensed orthopedists think is essential is lacking. Everyone in the hospital knows this, but you.
- And finally, there is a strong feeling that your x-ray department is understaffed and the services provided to the "bone man" are inadequate. On inquiry you find that the chief of x-ray may not be adding staff fast enough because of what it does to his own income. And everyone in the hospital knew this, too. Everyone but you.

Now all of the above is fairly typical of what you might find when you first start to dig deep into the situation. What started out as a rather isolated, and even simple, problem has turned into a rat's nest of intermingled "facts" and allegations.

At this point, people will say, "We can't talk about this." When you hear those words, you know you are getting close to something important. You are getting warm, and if you keep going, you will find an issue.

So instead of an official meeting in the hospital, you agree to a lunch downtown, near your office. Just you, another trustee, the chief executive of the hospital, and a couple of key physicians. At this meeting you begin, finally, to ask the right questions:

- How did this thing get so far without someone blowing the whistle?
- How is it possible for a situation like this to fester so long?
- What other storms are brewing that we don't know about?
- What's wrong with our communication around here?
- What blockages do we need to clear away?

And you agree to meet again, because now you know you are not dealing with a routine problem. You are dealing with an issue that demands resolution. And at the end of this whole process, I must warn you there is a high probability that you will discover the responsibility rests with you, the board of trustees.

The first point of all of this is that issue-oriented planning is different, tougher, and messier than financial planning. The issues are extremely hard to dig out and identify. They are rarely the same as you think at first. They are almost never what you are told. You have to dig.

The second point is that issues are often unspeakable. Often people can't bear the anguish of saying them out loud. Maybe it is a carryover from childhood, when it was awful to be branded a tattletale. Maybe it is because people don't want to disparage associates; it is an act of kindness to say nothing. Maybe, and most likely, most people in the hospital do not see the whole picture; they work in only a segment of it and do not see the whole pattern.

Whatever, keep in mind that it is your obligation to seek out the truth and act on it. The patients who use your hospital rely on you. Yes, it is fair to say to you, a board member, that lives depend on you. Lives are at stake. Lives are going to be saved or lost in your community, depending on the board's willingness and ability to tackle the issues.

Why Me?

This is the question trustees ask when the planning of the hospital's future is under discussion. Now that you have considered issue-oriented planning, the question has particular relevance — and poignancy.

You have an overwhelming feeling that with all these experts around you cannot contribute much. You look at the doctors in their white coats and say, "*They're* the ones who know all about health care. They should do it." And you look at the administrative staff and say, "*They're* the people with the training. Not only that, they're paid to do it." And you look at the old hands on the board, the ones who have been there for 20 years, and say, "*They're* the men and women with the vision and the experience. They can do it."

All of these people have a critical contribution to make. All are essential to the planning process. But they also may be a big part of the problem. Maybe they are the ones who got the hospital into its present sorry state.

As a trustee, you are the one person in the hospital who is neither so narrowly trained nor so thoroughly embedded in the present system that you can't see the whole institution in the context of the community it serves. Think of it: the one *generalist* around, the one person in the whole place who can ask naive questions without fear of appearing dumb, the one person who can demand that complex issues be explained simply so that you can understand — and thus everyone else will understand better.

You are the one person who can insist that the jargon and technical language of medicine, of the administrators (who are just as bad), and of the government agencies (who are worst of all) be put into plain-folks English. And that is to the benefit of all. When hospital people use language to impress one another, communication and understanding are the losers. You can and will always help sticky situations by improving communication, by playing the dummy who says repeatedly, "Put it in words I can understand."

You have other advantages. You are not suspected of monetary motivations. You are not going to make more money, no matter how a vote goes. You are something of a mystery — a businessman, a lawyer, a mother, or whatever, pouring energy and time into the hospital. You are respected for that. You are also respected for having an outside area of competence, for having experience that is new to and usually valued at the hospital.

So you have great strengths. You have something important to bring to the party: your own good head. Your inquiring naivete about medical things can also be a strength. It is simply invaluable in a situation where almost everyone looks at his own small corner of the problem and generalizes outward.

Your weakness (this is dealt with later) is your lack of information in a fast moving, immensely complex field. So your weakness is exactly what you thought it was.

But for now, think of yourself as a tower of strength, badly needed, and giving you particular value as you plan your hospital's future. You're the one who has the best chance to lead the effort, to come up with good answers to your hospital's problems. That's the answer to "Why me?"

But the main reason this book is aimed at trustees is a sequence of logic that runs like this:

- *Trustees are important to their hospitals.* Many trustees don't really believe it, but it is a fact that they are legally in power, legally responsible and accountable. Trustees have big-time responsibilities that cannot be delegated.
- *Trustees need more information about the health care process.* Trustees are generally bright and are knowledgeable about their own business affairs, but for the most part they do not know much about the complex business of providing health care. It is a highly regulated and technologically advanced industry. Trustees need to know about law and about medicine and medical gadgetry.
- *There are factions to be heard from and contended with.* Some of the best-fed egos in the country reside in hospitals. A hospital is not a unified environment, not an autocratically run enterprise.

- *The economics are tough.* Selling prices, which used to be established by the market, are now established by others outside the hospital.
- *The economic consequences of decisions made in hospitals are never "clean."* Some of the best decisions the hospital makes lose a ton of money, but they save lives. That's the problem: every decision is a trade-off between that which is medically desirable and that which is economically possible. This is the battleground. The situation isn't simple to begin with and, worse, it changes monthly, daily.
- *Trustees are part of the problem.* If you acknowledge that many trustees are not sufficiently informed about the issues or the mechanics of health care but that they have a large vote, then it is not a big jump in logic to conclude that they contribute to the problem rather than the solution.
- *Trustees can be bigger contributors to solutions.* Here's why: Doctors, nurses, administrators, government planners, and educators are all deeply enmeshed in their own small corners of the health care field, which is not only complex, but so big that no one person knows any more than a fragment. The health care field is sliced up and dispersed in so many directions that those who live inside it wrap their arms around just what they can see and comprehend and declare *that* to be the whole world. No one has a better chance to see it all and to see it in perspective than informed trustees. They came to the party with their outside experience and a detachment that is almost impossible for insiders to achieve. But note the use of the word *informed.* To be part of the solution, trustees need background and they need constant updating on the changing ground rules.

That is the logic that prompted this book for trustees. You can provide solutions. You can provide direction because you are in a unique position. And your hospital's long-range survival may very well depend on you. A lot of hospitals will be among the missing five years from now. A lot of people in your community are depending on you to see that *their* hospital is still there and functioning when they need it.

Long-Range Planning: The Time to Start Is Now

Most hospitals have been talking about long-range, or strategic, planning for years, but few have done much.

One reason they have done so little is that they confuse strategic planning with financial planning. This is common in other businesses also, particularly businesses dominated by financial types. They point to the deck of numbers that has been projected for the next five years and say, "See, long-range plans." That is not long-range planning, but only a projection of the number trends. It leaves out consideration of the things your hospital *could* be or *ought* to be. It leaves out consideration of alternatives, even including closing down forever (yes, sometime in your planning process you must appraise that possibility).

In short, financial planning just pushes your current experience ahead. The basic premise is whatever you are doing now is what you will be doing tomorrow. Strategic planning, on the other hand, can, and often does, lead to change. It can change part of the enterprise or redirect it entirely.

Another reason why hospitals have done so little strategic planning is they don't know how. They don't know where to begin, and, once started, how to proceed. Maybe this is because hospitals are populated by many highly trained people — the doctors and the administrators — who are uncomfortable without the regimens, disciplines, and guidelines they work within all the time. At this time long-range planning is more of an art form than a science, and it is a bruising process.

Well, here you are. No long-range plans. In crisis. Events closing in on you. Do you know the proper time to get started on planning at your hospital? There is only one time. *Now.* As imperfect, as unready, as untrained as you are, the perfect time to start is now. Otherwise you will discover two years down the road that you are still "getting ready," that your competitors are making headway, and that some of your options have been closed off by inaction.

Start. Now. Get going.

Getting the Long-Range Planning Committee Organized

Committees, and committee meetings, are everyone's curse. For your purposes, however, it is the way to go. What you want at the other end of the process is consensus, everyone moving in the same direction, everyone working toward the common good. You want the hatchets buried—and in some place other than in one another's skulls.

Call it a task force, or any other name, it is still a committee, with all the problems and advantages inherent and intact. Here is what you need:

- *Size.* Size is important. The committee should number between 10 and 15. Any fewer than 7 won't produce the right dynamics. Any more than 15 and the flow and discussion of ideas—communication—will be lost. People start to make speeches; others fail to listen; some hide and never speak.
- *Representation.* All the key-player groups must be represented. There absolutely must be substantial representation from the medical staff and from the board. The chief executive officer and one or two from the CEO's staff must be included. You can also have some others, depending on their personalities and qualifications and on the needs of your hospital.
- *Medical staff.* Be sure that the doctors who are selected have maximum credibility. If there are opposing camps (and it is almost certain that there are, as all medical staffs numbering more than two are divided into factions), be absolutely sure that all camps

are represented. Pick doctors who have much at stake at your hospital and who have proven to be effective workers on staff committees. Do not pick doctors just because they are friendly, unless they have the respect of the medical staff. Give doctors a majority, so there is no question at the implementation stage about whose plan this is.

- *The board.* Every board of trustees is composed of a mix of the highly motivated, who are the workers, and the attendees, who show up at the meetings, fill a seat, but do not make their presence felt in any other way. *Pick workers.* You might have a choice of lawyers, self-employed people, homemakers, and executives from big corporations. *Go for at least two big-company executives if you have them.* They are accustomed to the life and realities of the political jungle of corporations. They will understand the hospital's organizational complexities better than most others. Lawyers and persons who work in small professional offices do not generally have much appreciation for the political subtleties of hospital organization.

- *Brains.* If your board is typical, you will have the normal frequency curve of brainpower to pick from. *Go for the bright ones.* Brainpower is the one irreplaceable ingredient on the committee.

- *Administration.* The chief executive officer of the hospital must be on the committee, deeply involved in every meeting. If you were thinking of withholding anything from him, you'd be making a mistake. In addition, you and the CEO may want one of his key lieutenants. It is essential that the hospital's administration be effectively represented, for these three reasons: The administration must be seen by the medical staff as a partner, an important equal in the fight for the hospital's survival. The administration will carry much of the load in the action phase of planning. The administration will carry much of the fact-gathering burden of the planning process.

- *Chairman.* The chairman must be one of the members of the board, but should *not* be the chairman of the board. The chairman can, and should, be impartial — a neutral, a seeker of great truths. Doctors and administrators have a tough time posing as neutrals; someone is always convinced they have ulterior motives. The chairman should be clear thinking, have good communication skills, and be adept at running meetings.

- *Leadership style.* The chairman has a tough job. He must be sure every faction is heard, even when his own biases are challenged. He must milk ideas from the group and subdue his own ideas, recognizing that the group has a much higher sense of ownership for an idea that it produces than for one the chairman produces. Above all, the chairman must keep the group from veering off the subject. The committee members will exhibit an unerring skill in caroming off just as an issue is about to be exposed and discussed. The chairman must bring them back. He must not yield when someone says, "We need more data," "We must start research," or "It is time to adjourn." He must go for the jugular when an issue is finally unearthed and demand that the group argue it through.

- *Consultants.* You should not use consultants to do your planning for you, but it is OK to use them as resources, sounding boards, or aides. The plan that emerges, however, must be the committee's — an original, authored by your hospital, and, above all, *believed* by your key people. If it is thought to be authored by consultants, it will not have the commitment needed to get action.

- *Action.* Perhaps the message is beginning to come through, now that the kind of planning being recommended is probably quite different from what you have experienced at your hospital. What you are after is results, action, all of the major issues out in the open being discussed and argued about, even though it is painful, so that resolution can be achieved. At the end of the process, things should be happening. Change should be visible. You should know where you are headed. Action, not a thick report, is your objective.

The Long-Range Planning Committee's Charge

One hospital has labeled the long-range planning committee of its board the Challenge Committee. Whatever its name, the committee should not begin work until its function has been agreed upon. Here is a suggestion for the charge:

> The long-range planning committee shall make recommendations for long-range goals and objectives for the hospital. It shall attempt to be aware of all developments in the health care field and trends in society and to interpret the effect of these developments and trends on the hospital. A principal function of the committee shall be the development of a written statement describing the hospital's specific role in the community in relation to all other health care facilities. The long-range planning committee shall recommend a strategy for the hospital to pursue and shall monitor the hospital's progress in achieving it. The chief executive officer of the hospital shall be on the committee, and the hospital administrative staff, under the CEO's direction, shall assist the committee in its work. There shall be at least two members of the medical staff on the committee.

This charge will serve as a model and give you a start on writing your own. Use it also as a resolution to modify the bylaws of your hospital in order to give the committee official status.

Now let's examine the charge. It makes clear that the long-range planning committee derives its authority from the board of trustees. That means that, like any other board committee, it is responsible to the full board and reports back to it.

The committee's time frame is explicitly long range. It should stay out of current operations and the administrator's hair and out of the way of the other board committees, which are working on current business most of the time.

The committee's job is to consider major issues of all sorts, major projects, and priorities, and to make recommendations to the board. Major expenditures should usually be considered first by this committee and next by the finance committee.

The charge implies that the committee has the further duties and obligations to:

- Develop a framework for orderly decision making, through a defined community role called the mission statement, a set of long-term goals and objectives, a strategy for achievement, and a timetable for recommended progress.
- Ensure that all recommendations coming from this and other committees fit within the hospital's defined role, facilitate achievement of its goals and objectives, and follow the long-range plan. It is a continuing obligation of the committee to keep the hospital on course with its plan (or strategy) or to change the plan as new facts and conditions dictate.
- Develop a sense of priorities in its examination of issues and projects so that the hospital's limited resources of time and money are spent on those projects that take it the furthest in achieving its defined role in the community.
- Act as a vehicle for good communication among the board, the medical staff, and the administration.

That is the charge the long-range planning committee needs from the board to get started.

The Process Is Important

The process is more than important; it is the whole ball game. You are going after results, change, not just a written document. That is why the process, the meetings you hold, the people you involve, the way you involve them, the pain, the arguments, and the hard work of thinking are all so important.

Here is the rule, and it is dogma: The 25 percent plan that gets 100 percent commitment is a winner; the 100 percent plan that gets 25 percent commitment is a loser.

What does that mean? It means that neither the administrator, nor the chairman of the board, nor the consultant you hire hands out a plan and asks everyone to agree. That is a guaranteed way to eliminate involvement, to cut off exchange of information, discussion, argument, and exposing of issues. It means that what you are after is consensus, agreement on the approach. The leaders should be ready to act in concert. Consensus can be achieved only when the ideas emerge from the group itself. They cannot be imposed by one doctor, one president, one chairman of the board, or one planner.

Achieving consensus also means that hard work is part of the process. Without it you will not get good ideas, understanding of the issues and commitment, and you will not get action. What you *will* get is a lot of people looking at their watches and, in the end, a five-pound plan in a stiff-cover, gold-leaf-inscribed volume that no one will ever read or act on. A total waste of time. If the objective of your planning is to minimize effort, to avoid arguments, to lay off the work on others, to maintain the status quo, then you should state that up front and forget about planning. You won't get meaningful results anyway.

So let's assume your group is ready to work, ready to dig in. Here are some nuts-and-bolts techniques for you to use:

- *Meet in the right room.* Meet in a room that is not too big, or the group will feel intimidated. Arrange comfortable chairs in an arch, crescent, or U shape, so that everyone can look directly at everyone else. The leader should be in the opening, where he can have eye contact with every member. Under no circumstances should you meet in the hospital boardroom. It is the wrong environment: too comfortable for the board members, too uncomfortable for the doctors. In fact, it is best if you get out of the hospital and meet in a good conference facility.

- *Arrange meetings of the right length.* The best choice is an overnight meeting. Start at 2 p.m. on day one, stop for dinner from 5:30 to 7 p.m., resume and continue to about 9:30 p.m. Start day two with breakfast and end at 5 p.m. The minimum length for a meeting should be four hours; six or seven hours is better. Don't meet for longer than seven hours no matter what, because if you do continue meeting, you won't get anything done.

- *Have the right facilities.* They should be simple: comfortable chairs and side tables for coffee cups. *Do not have a big board table.* Board tables inhibit discussion, invite speeches, and create a noninnovative environment. Also, do not have phones or electronic pages in the meeting room. Make coffee available from the start of the meeting, and have cold drinks available in the afternoon. Lunches should be light: cold cuts and salads, for example. Don't put your workers to sleep with heavy meals. You will need two large easels (about 24 inches by 36 inches) for chart paper, flow pens, a supply of push pins, and masking tape.

- *Use the easel charts constantly.* The charts are an important part of the process. The discussion leader or planning chairman is the person to run them. Don't ever use handouts except as resource material. The leader should record the meeting on the charts as it progresses, putting down what he hears as it is said. This is a critical part of the process and accomplishes several things simultaneously:
  - It helps learning, because the leader reinforces what is said by writing it on the chart at the front of the room.
  - It makes people responsible for what they have said. Frequently, in heat, some great truths emerge, as do some irresponsible things. The technique of writing everything down lets speakers amend, or others attack, what has been said.

—It focuses the attention of all participants on the same issue; it keeps the group together.
—It allows ideas to be stored on paper as the group moves on to other subjects. Simply rip the sheet off the pad and put it on the wall; you can return to it later.
—It records the meeting, so good ideas aren't lost. Later the gems can be extracted from material in the piles of charts.

- *Read the body language.* If you have assembled a planning group of 12, you will discover some who are loquacious, some who don't want to say anything, some who are uptight, some who are cynical, and some who are uninformed but willing. The leader's job is to be sure that all of these persons are heard and to register their views. This is where body signals come in. When Dr. A is speaking and Dr. B is wearing a frown, the leader must be sure to call on Dr. B; she won't volunteer. When board member C is spouting his theories and member D looks as though he is going to cloud up and rain, the leader should be sure to get member D to talk.
- *Keep everyone involved and alert.* The leader should keep monitoring the group and keep drawing the members out: "Do you agree with that?" "Why are you squirming in your chair while Ed speaks?" If the group has struck on an important point but two or three persons are monopolizing the meeting, the leader should stop the process: "We're going to hear from the others on this. Starting on my left, what do you think?" If the group has been at it for a few hours and looks exhausted, the leader should break off the meeting for 10 minutes: "We're hung up on this one. Let's stop here. Get out of the room, take a walk, and be back in 10 minutes."

These are simple approaches, proven over years of planning experience, designed to help you get into the process. Remember, the process generates the action. The documents you will ultimately produce do not. Remember that what you are after is consensus and commitment, and you get it through involvement in the process.

Outline of the Plan

The long-range planning committee's final presentation to the board of trustees and the medical staff is very likely going to follow an outline that looks something like this:

Facts about our hospital

- Historical background: founding, major additions, major changes in ownership or in health care role
- Trended statistical data for the past 10 years, showing utilization by major departments, room rates, expenditures, income
- Current medical staff data
- Trade area served (the geographic area and the people who live in it)
- Data on competitive facilities in the area

Trends, and where they appear to be taking us

- Society
- Government
- Medical developments
- Health care
- Competitive plans
- The hospital's own trends projected ahead five years on the assumption of no change
- The hospital's own trends projected ahead five years on the assumption of changes in society, government, medical developments, and health care

The stated role of the hospital (also called the mission statement)

- As it is (or is not) now written

- As it should be written, recognizing all the facts, problems, strengths, and weaknesses we know about
- Compared with the stated role of other nearby institutions

The strengths of the hospital: what we've got to build on in achieving our ambitions in the next 5 to 10 years

- Medical staff
- Nursing staff
- Facilities
- Reputation
- Trade area
- Management
- Board
- Other

The issues to be addressed: the problems we must solve if we are to succeed in our mission in the next 5 to 10 years

- Medical staff
- Nursing staff
- Facilities
- Reputation
- Management
- Board
- Relationships with other health care facilities
- Other

Alternative planning solutions for the next 5 to 10 years

- Ideas that might solve the problems
- Each alternative assessed for cost impact
- Each alternative assessed for potential results

Recommended course of action for the next 5 to 10 years: timing and action

- Who will do what, and when
- Who must approve
- What costs will be incurred
- What savings will be made
- What results are expected, and when

This outline is classic and proven. Use it as the working structure for the planning effort for your hospital. This is one area in which you should not be innovative; don't reinvent the wheel.

Time Out: Who Is Doing All the Work?

Now is probably the time to remind you that:

- You are working on a committee that reports to the board of trustees. It does not have a life of its own.
- The committee was carefully chosen to represent the important factions and viewpoints of the hospital and consists of board members, physicians, and key management personnel from the hospital. Each member has communication responsibilities.
- The committee will delegate work to the hospital staff: occasionally to individual physicians, board members, or another committee, but mostly to the management staff of the hospital.

If the committee is working effectively, you will meet often, at least twice a month and maybe once a week. You will find that these are some of the most frustrating meetings you are involved with; people getting upset, mad, hollering. The meetings will be long. In fact, there will probably be a few all-day meetings.

If you are working effectively, you will feel that, for the first time, you are really beginning to grasp what makes the wheels go around, who is doing what to whom, and why you are experiencing anxieties. In short, being on the long-range planning committee is a learning process, and everyone on the committee will know he has been somewhere and done something and will be set to develop some answers.

So who is doing all the work? You are doing a lot of it. But the hospital staff should be doing the digging for the committee, coming up with the information it needs in order to function.

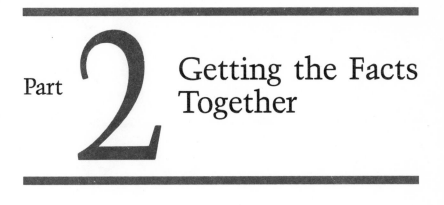

Part **2** Getting the Facts
Together

Digging for Facts: The Nuts and Bolts of Planning

This book is addressed to survival, to helping you ensure the continuation of your hospital. Why, then, stress so pedestrian an idea as digging for facts? Precisely because this is where most hospital planning has fallen apart. Most hospital planning, including that done by government agencies and that being done by some of the business consortiums, has begun with answers instead of questions. That is why so much planning effort has proven fruitless.

One of the most effective approaches to planning is to steadfastly identify missing information and relentlessly dig for facts. (In this connection, the outline beginning on page 34 is useful.) Here are some steps to follow in bringing facts to light:

- Survival starts here, with the facts of the situation. Don't even dream about working on solutions until your planning committee has the facts under control: discovered, organized, and understood. There is an important reason why your planning committee should be relentlessly digging for facts. If you push for facts long enough, great truths will emerge and solutions to the hospital's problems will present themselves.
- Because the objective of planning is to anticipate the future and accommodate the surprises that the future holds, you must think seriously about trends. Start by projecting the hospital's statistical data. When you do this, you are saying, in effect, "If we do nothing to modify our behavior, if the social climate remains constant, if our competitors stand still, and if no one comes up with a medical breakthrough, this is what we expect." If your hospital

is simply projecting present numbers, you are working on the premise that you will be living in a change-free environment, and if that is so, your hospital does not deserve to survive. You must accommodate the trends of society, government, medicine, and technology in your planning for the future.

- State a clear mission for your hospital. The mission statement is the job description of your hospital stated in community terms, and it considers the community's needs, the hospital's medical capabilities, and the hospital's financial ability to serve. The statement is a tool designed to communicate what the hospital stands for. It is the beginning point of discipline that will allow you to sensibly appraise requests for money, new equipment, new staff, and new facilities. The mission statement is the beginning of your plan.

These three steps—digging for the facts, understanding and adjusting for the trends, and developing a mission statement—represent the essential process of planning your hospital's survival.

The Patient Is a Customer

Many of the people who staff hospitals have social service leanings. They want to help others. They want to be loved. They want to be positioned out of and above the grind of commerce. But that is an impossible stance to maintain at a time when newspapers are packed full of stories about nurses going on strike, doctors joining unions, and room rates brushing up against $1,000 per day in some hospitals. The notion that all who work at the hospital do it only for the love of their fellow human beings no longer has credibility in our society, and the image of the hospital as a place of charity has about had it.

That is why the word *customer*, instead of *patient*, appears in this book. It is time to think about those terms, because the hospital and its patients are drifting apart, and there is frustration on both sides. As a planner, you must concern yourself with this state of affairs.

The word *patient* has connotations that probably are at the heart of much distress and friction that exist between health care professionals and the people who go to hospitals for help.

Consider these statements:

- A patient is someone I help.
- A patient is often in a horizontal position.
- A patient is someone to be cared for.
- A patient is often seated or supine when I talk to him. I am standing, so the patient looks up at me and I look down at him.
- A patient is someone who looks to me for life, and I help him because I am good.
- A patient is someone I stick with needles to make him well.
- A patient is someone I talk to with big words.
- A patient is someone who, were he as smart as I am, would be a doctor or a nurse or a trustee, too.

- A patient waits, well, *patiently*, in my office because I am busy and important.

Patient implies subordinate and dependent. It seems also to imply, "I am helping you. When I treat you, it is my little contribution to your well-being. Please remember to thank me. Be grateful. Act like a patient."

That's the problem. If you are the patient who has just stepped up to the window in the business office of your hospital and written a check for $3,000 to cover a five-day hospital stay, you do not feel like a patient. You do not feel grateful. You do not feel like the lucky recipient of the loving care the doctors, the nurses, and the hospital have provided. No, you feel like a customer. You feel as though you have just paid a bundle for those services. You do not feel as though you owe anyone excessive gratitude, and that is where the rub comes in. That patients are more demanding and more militant in direct relationship to increasing hospital costs is just about fact 1 for you to understand in planning the hospital's future.

The patient *is* a customer. Many hospital people have a hard time swallowing this fact, so perhaps those of you on the board who make your livelihood in commercial endeavors can help the hospital people over the hump. Help them to think there is nothing quite so wonderful as a customer. If you can teach them to value a customer, that it is *they* who must learn to say "Thank you," you can reduce much of the tension that is blocking the road to effective care.

Understanding
the Customer Base

Hospitals have trade areas, much like department stores. You need to understand the limits of your hospital's trade (or service) area, what is going on there, and what is likely to happen in the future.

Successful department stores know the customers of their trade area better than unsuccessful stores. Successful stores know where their customers live, how old they are, how they live, where they wished they lived, how they spend their time, and how they spend their money. The customers are more than a source of money; they are a source of fascination. Great stores never cease trying to understand their customers. That's one of the keys to their greatness.

Because hospitals can learn much from the merchants, this chapter asks you to be talented and artful borrowers of facts and materials already in existence in your community:

- *Start with a map.* Mark on it the location of your hospital and every other hospital with whom you compete for patients, that is, customers. The word *compete* is deliberate. Survival demands that you use such language and not smother reality by the use of words like *share.* You do not share customers; you compete for them. And this map begins to show you a crude sort of reality about your hospital.
- *Now put the customers on the map.* Learn how government planners do this. Shade the areas to show dense pockets of population. Your hospital, of course, does not serve geographic areas; it serves concentrations of populations. Still, you want to look at the wide open spaces, too. If your hospital is in a small town

in Nebraska, the presence of 10,000 acres of adjacent farmland may not indicate much in terms of population. But if your hospital is in Houston, a 1,000-acre ranch a mile away probably means you are about to be serving a population explosion.

- *Now put the natural barriers on the map.* Worry about these. If your hospital is only a mile away from 200,000 people but that mile happens to be across a river and the nearest bridge is five miles away, that's different from one mile across land. Railroads are barriers, as are canals, creeks, and bayous. Airports, golf courses, military bases, and stockyards are barriers. Superhighways are big barriers. County lines and state lines are usually barriers. The point is that you don't just draw concentric circles around the hospital to understand the trade area.
- *Study patient/customer records.* Put a pin on the map for every customer admitted in a month. This usually turns up some surprises that should be explained. Explaining them is a principal source of clues for planners.

Mapping out your trade area is the beginning. As you do this, you will undoubtedly find some unexpected phenomena. Yet you would do well to go beyond these studies to another technique. The analogy of the department store is worth a return visit. Careful examination shows some interesting things going on. First of all, you discover that the store really is a collection of departments, each of which attracts its own kind of customers.

For example:

- The furniture department might be so good that it draws people from 100 miles away.
- The pharmacy department, on the other hand, might serve principally the needs of the employees who work in the store, so its draw is only about 300 feet.
- The men's suit department might draw only from professional and business people who work within five miles of the store.
- The better dresses department might draw customers a distance of 35 miles.
- Women's hosiery draws only working women within walking distance.

Now, if you tossed all these departments into one basket, you could come up with some of the world's most meaningless statistics, something like "Our store draws 70 percent of its business from a trading radius of 5 miles." The statement means nothing. It shows no strengths to build on and no departments that need remedial action. A figure that takes the average of all customers doesn't tell you much. So study your hospital by the following method. Record a useful sample of your customers in the configuration shown below.

Distance between Hospital and Customers' Homes

Department	Percentage of Customers		
	0-5 Miles	5-10 Miles	Over 10 Miles
Medicine			
Surgery			
Ob-Gyn			
Psychiatry			
Other			

You can make this study in any number of ways. For example, substitute mileage ranges that fit your trade area or use departmental divisions that suit your hospital.

Yours is a true community hospital if your figures look something like this:

Distance between Loving Arms Hospital and Customers' Homes

Department	Percentage of Customers		
	0-5 Miles	5-10 Miles	Over 10 Miles
Medicine	65	30	5
Surgery	60	30	10
Ob-Gyn	70	25	5
Psychiatry	55	30	15

In this example, most of the customers have come from the immediate area of the hospital; only a trickle has come farther than 10 miles. That is the way the figures for a true community hospital usually look.

Now look at the figures for another hospital:

Distance between Tender Care Hospital and Customers' Homes

Department	Percentage of Customers		
	0-5 Miles	5-10 Miles	Over 10 Miles
Medicine	60	20	20
Surgery	40	30	30
Ob-Gyn	85	10	5
Psychiatry	30	40	30

You would read these figures like this:

- Your medical admissions look like a community hospital in action, although 40 percent of customers coming from beyond the five-mile range might mean that some specialists on staff are attracting these customers.
- Your surgeons are getting referrals from a wide area; you should look with interest at what they are doing. Maybe you have a strength to build on. Maybe, on the other hand, you are at risk, if you have an older surgeon of renown who is responsible for drawing those referrals. Either way, the figures for surgery invite a searching look.
- Ob-Gyn looks like a straightforward community hospital situation, but when the planners start grading your hospital (categorization), will you lose out to a higher-ranked hospital? A worry.
- Your psychiatric unit is serving a regional need.

The point of these examples is that the examination of your hospital's trade, or service, areas by department is the real beginning of an understanding of your total customer trading area.

Here are the critical questions that should be asked and answered concerning the next 5 to 10 years:

- Will your trade area shrink or grow?
- Will the population in the area shrink, grow, or be stable?
- Will the population get younger or older?
- Will the population change ethnically?

- Will new barriers (like highways) be introduced and change the traffic pattern?

You should develop answers to all those questions before proceeding to develop your plan. You need the answers as input to your planning meetings.

Here is where you can go for basic information:

- Power companies
- Telephone companies
- Major retailers
- Planning agencies
- Banks
- Chambers of commerce

A word of caution: Don't accept what you get from these sources as totally reliable. They, too, can be wrong. Think about the data you get and modify them according to your own thinking and knowledge.

Tuning In on the Community

The hospital administration must have a good feeling for what is going on around the hospital; it must be in touch on an ongoing basis with the immediate neighborhood and the customers who live there. If your hospital is to be counted among the survivors years from now, one of the reasons will be that you developed sensitive listening posts in the community.

Many hospital board members do not have a clue about the hospital community, because they do not live near the hospital they serve. City hospitals often are located in the old part of town; but the trustees, administrative staff, doctors, and nurses often live in the suburbs. It is only the custodial staff who reside in the community in which the hospital is located and who become the hospital's links to the community, the hospital's eyes and ears *and* spokesmen and spokeswomen.

Therefore you need to develop an orderly flow of information about the population your hospital serves. You must know what your customers have on their minds. If you are not trying diligently to learn what your customers want, you are not behaving responsibly as a trustee of a big community asset, that is, your hospital. If you have not taken the time to listen, you cannot spend big chunks of money in the community without running severe risks.

A principal reason so many hospitals have been zapped by the political process rests right here: the politicians were more sensitive to what the customers were saying than were the hospitals. The message that customers were saying something serious still hasn't reached many members of hospital boards. The politicians heard it; they didn't.

Here are three things you should do on an ongoing basis. It is unlikely you are doing any of them systematically, so start now, as you crank up the planning process at your hospital.

Conduct Consumer Attitude Research

Most hospitals send questionnaires to some of their patients (rate our food service, nursing care, and so forth). That is not enough. Hire a competent consumer research firm to determine what people think of you, what their attitudes or perceptions are. The survey should be done every year so that you can:

- Measure your progress
- Determine how patients view you
- Learn how the patients of *other* hospitals perceive you
- Compare your "profile" with that of hospitals near you.

This study shows the areas in which your hospital has shortcomings that need to be corrected. The follow-up annual questionnaire tells you if you are making progress. This is a methodical approach to finding out what your customers have on their minds and whether you are responding to these needs. It is how professional marketers make sure they know what is going on "out there." It is how they attempt to keep surprises to a minimum. Hospitals can learn from them.

I recommend that *all* hospitals use marketing research techniques on a consistent basis. The big marketing companies learned long ago that personal knowledge of a market is very often the most dangerous information you have, simply because so often it is wrong. So gather information systematically; use professionals.

Reverse Your Approach with Civic Clubs

Hospital trustees and administrators have been fond of telling the hospital's story at a Lions International Club or a Rotary Club lunch, for example. That is probably useful. However, perhaps the hospital would do better if it were to listen instead of talk. It is easy to forget that communication must be a two-way process and that you may have been transmitting but not receiving. So the next time you go to the civic club to tell the story, take these steps beforehand:

- Send the club president enough copies of a letter to mail to the club's membership three weeks before you participate in the program. The letter should ask the recipients to fill out and return a letter that follows the outline on the next page.
- When the letters are returned, analyze the results and build your talk around the problems that are mentioned.

If you or the administrator of your hospital does this a half-dozen times in the year, you will discover that patterns emerge. These are

```
┌─────────────────────────────────────────────────────────────┐
│                                                             │
│   Dear (Hospital)                                           │
│                                                             │
│     The three things I like best about your hospital are:   │
│                                                             │
│                                                             │
│        1. _____  │
│                                                             │
│        2. _____  │
│                                                             │
│        3. _____  │
│                                                             │
│                                                             │
│     The three things I dislike most about your hospital are:│
│                                                             │
│                                                             │
│        1. _____  │
│                                                             │
│        2. _____  │
│                                                             │
│        3. _____  │
│                                                             │
│                                                             │
│        _____                         │
│     Signed (If you wish to do so)                           │
│                                                             │
└─────────────────────────────────────────────────────────────┘
```

a consensus of concerns for you to listen to and real problems for you to address. You will also discover that the simple act of listening begins to defuse the problems. A hospital that conspicuously listens well is hard to dislike.

Conduct Focus-Group Interviews

This is a technique for finding out what the right questions are. Eight or 10 persons are brought together by a group leader who is skilled at getting people to interact. (Focus-group interviews, like most consumer research, should be conducted by professionals.) In two hours, eight individuals can cover a lot of territory and give you many insights.

There is another use: Have your planning committee listen to a focus group discuss your hospital. The experience will be a great deflator of pompous self-impressions and a great beginning to understanding your problems.

Tuning in on the community, getting close to what customers want and don't want, is part of the survival process. The three ideas proposed here will help you get in touch and stay in touch.

Looking at the Competition

Until just a few years ago, it was considered gauche in the hospital world to refer to other health care institutions as competitors. That was and is unfortunate, because the concept of competition is a valuable one. Hospitals that survive are likely to use the word *competition* often. Although it is possible for competition to be carried too far, I know of no single instance where it has been carried far enough.

If your planning committee doesn't understand your hospital's competitors, it will make some poor decisions. Failure to understand competitors — their strategies, what they are good at, what they are building, and where they are going — has probably led the health care industry to more wasted capital expenditures than any other single cause. Understanding competitors is important to your hospital's survival; it is one way by which you can ensure that your limited resources are spent wisely and are not blown on simply matching the competition.

Use a matrix to study your competition. Start with a study of beds as shown on the following page.

The breakdown of the numbers and types of beds that you use in your matrix depends on your hospital. For instance, if you have a drug treatment facility, you will want to know how many similar beds there are in other facilities. For many hospitals, this leads to an important discovery: they have competitors they don't ordinarily think of — nursing homes, alcoholism treatment centers, specialized hospitals in far-off places, clinics, and so forth.

The matrix is the A in the ABCs of understanding your competitors. If you haven't discovered and listed about 10 competitors whose facilities your specific community uses, you probably haven't dug deep enough. If your hospital is located in a major city, you should be able

Total Number of Beds

	Percentage of Beds		
Type of Bed	Your Hospital	Tender Care Hospital	Loving Arms Hospital
Medical			
Surgical			
Ob-Gyn			
Bassinets			
Psychiatric			
Chemical dependency			
Alcoholism			
Extended care			
Nursing home			
All other open			
Closed			
Other			

to list about 20 directly competitive facilities. More than half of those will not come readily to mind. You will have to dig for them.

Here are examples of what you can discover:

- If your 200-bed hospital has a 20-bed psychiatric unit that is using only 50 percent of its capacity, the reason may be a 100-bed psychiatric unit in a medical school 35 miles away that is operating at 90 percent capacity.
- If your 20-bed intermediate care nursing unit is running at 100 percent capacity, it may be because there is no similar, licensed institution in your area.
- If your 10-bed Ob-Gyn department is running with only 2 or 3 beds utilized, you may discover eight other places also running at 20 or 30 percent capacity.

Simple bed counts are where you start the process of understanding competitors. The next step is to repeat the matrix, but this time plug in your competitors' utilization rates for the most recent year. Why should you look at their utilization rates? The rates tell you where your competitors' strengths and weaknesses are. For example:

Utilization of Beds

Type of Bed	Percentage of Beds		
	Your Hospital	Tender Care Hospital	Loving Arms Hospital
Medical	84	85	70
Surgical	95	95	65
Ob-Gyn	60	40	40
Psychiatric	60	30	100

Some facts now jump at you:

- Loving Arms Hospital has strength in psychiatry but is not strong in surgery or medical utilization.
- Tender Care Hospital might be interested in closing out both psychiatric and Ob-Gyn beds, whereas it is strong in medical and surgical services.
- Although your hospital leads only in Ob-Gyn, it probably has the greatest all-around strength.

You can correctly assume that there is concern about overall occupancy at each of these hospitals. You can also assume that:

- Loving Arms Hospital is thinking about converting beds to psychiatric use (expansion) and is perhaps giving careful thought to Ob-Gyn.
- Tender Care Hospital's surgical department appears to be bursting at the seams. You can see a new operating suite coming up and possibly the conversion to surgical use of some unused beds.

Thus, by means of these simple matrixes, you are beginning to understand your competitors in some depth. You now know who they are and what their strengths and weaknesses are. By projecting yourself into their shoes, you also should have a fair idea of their plans for the future.

Where do you get the data on your competitors? You ask them for it. Most hospitals quite readily exchange such data. Many hospitals publish the figures in their annual reports. And finally, you can find the data in the appropriate planning agencies.

Understanding and sizing up your competitors and assessing their strengths and weaknesses accurately are critical to the survival of your hospital and essential for your community. They are key ways by which you will avoid squandering the hospital's resources, just as one of the ways by which Colgate and Lever avoid destroying themselves is by studying Proctor and Gamble.

That is just the start, however. Real understanding of competitors' strengths and weaknesses can only be gained with research among the customers of each hospital. You need to know why they prefer another hospital before you can come to grips with your hospital's weaknesses.

What customers think of you and your competitors today is a very accurate predictor of the hospital they will go to when the need arises tomorrow.* In short, you can come close to predicting your volume and the volume of competitors on the basis of customer preference.

So, understanding competitors means understanding how customers rate them.

---

*For a more thorough examination of the process customers use in selecting hospitals, see *Marketing Your Hospital: A Strategy for Survival*, by Norman H. McMillan (Chicago: American Hospital Association, 1981).

Interinstitutional Relationships

Throughout the past 10 or 15 years, government has urged hospitals to work more effectively with other agencies in the community. This is a promising idea. It could lead to higher quality care in some of the secondary health care facilities such as nursing homes, and it could help the economics of hospitals, although neither of these conclusions is certain.

When your hospital begins planning, some of the questions you should ask are, "What agencies do we work with?" "What other health care facilities do we exchange information with?" "Who are the people we help?" "How do we work together to lower costs?"

Before you start anything new, you should take stock of where you are. There is a high probability you already are involved in more working relationships with other health care institutions than you realize. These liaisons probably run the gamut from totally informal arrangements to joint ownership of facilities.

Through a little digging, one hospital's planning committee developed a list of working relationships the hospital had established with other health care facilities. Here are excerpts from their list:

- Joint ownership of a laundry with four other hospitals in the city
- Purchase of linen for a nursing home in the neighborhood
- Participation in a tumor registry with another hospital
- Rental of time on a computer that belongs to an insurance company
- Purchase of computer cardiac services from a medical clinic
- Shared teaching programs with a university medical school

- Group purchase of drugs with 13 other hospitals
- Operation with three other hospitals of a school of anesthesiology

The only surprise, and it *was* a surprise to everyone, was the length of the list: 13 sharing arrangements all in place and functioning routinely.

Now the second step. Make another matrix in which you list all the relationships you have with other institutions. The matrix should look like this:

Working Relationships with Other Hospitals

Activity	Hospital A	Hospital B	Hospital C	Hospital D	Hospital E
1	•	•	•	•	•
2	•			•	
3		•			
4			•		
5		•			
6	•	•	•		
7					
8	•	•		•	•
9		•			
10		•			

The matrix shows an actual example, and in this instance the planning committee discovered something of extreme interest: the hospital was pursuing a strategy of alliance with Hospital B *without knowing it*. Low-level to medium-level linkages had been established all over the hospital, department by department. Without planning, or as one trustee commented, "Untouched by human thought," substantial alliances had been created. This is one reason why you must look at what is going on. You may get a pleasant surprise, as this hospital did.

The right way to start is by defining what kind of institution your hospital intends to be. Only after you've done that can you figure out with whom you should make your alliances. Be sure you get legal advice before proceeding, as there are some topics, such as cutting or allocation of services, that hospitals simply *cannot* get together and talk about.

An important generality that probably has not yet been fully grasped is that health care is no longer just the art of healing the sick or preventing the well from getting ill. To provide health care effectively now requires a hospital to appreciate that it is deeply enmeshed in politics. It is no longer possible for a hospital to provide good health care without having good relationships with various government agencies, planners, and politicians.

The conclusions seem inevitable. First, your hospital must take steps to make itself a more effective political force in the community. This means learning what the community's political wants and needs are and responding to them. Your hospital will also have to find ways to accommodate probably greater expenditures of money and manpower to achieve these aims.

A further conclusion seems equally inevitable. Your hospital will speak more effectively, get a bigger hearing, if it represents a lot of votes rather than a few votes. So you can anticipate the formation of coalitions in health care partly for good sound health care reasons, but mostly for power-block reasons. Obviously 5,000 beds, representing the efforts of 10,000 doctors, nurses, and employees, speak louder and are heard more clearly than 100 beds ever will be.

The message is clear, and your hospital should address it: politics, politicians, and bureaucrats are very much more important to you now than they were in the past. Before your hospital undertakes backing political candidates or influencing legislation, it will, of course, need sound legal advice to make sure that the proposed activities are lawful under both state and federal law, will not jeopardize any federal tax exemption, and otherwise will not create any new legal problems.

If a planning agency exists in your area, you should get to know its staff well. If you have a coalition of business firms in your community that is getting under way to see if it cannot help control health care costs, obviously you want to be involved to the extent possible.

It probably also makes sense to form strong alliances with other health care institutions. What kind should they be? The answer is, it depends. It depends almost entirely on how you see the future, on what you have defined as your role in the community. There is no point in your developing miscellaneous relationships with alcoholism and drug treatment centers, for instance, if your own ambitions do not move you in that direction. On the other hand, if you have a very strong record and capability as a trauma center, you might want to be sure that highway signs are adequate to direct people in need to your hospital.

So before you rush off to form miscellaneous relationships with other health care facilities, take step 1: figure out what your mission is for the next 5 to 10 years.

Making Utilization Figures Talk

The utilization rate is to the hospital what the Dow Jones is to the stock market. What you as a trustee must understand is that this figure is a composite of everything that goes on in your hospital. It is a measure of how many beds are filled, and that is a reliable economic indicator. Like the Dow Jones, the higher the figure, the better it is.

Utilization is always expressed as a percentage. If you have 100 beds and 82 was the average number filled in January, your January utilization was 82 percent. The 82 percent figure means several simple things:

- It is a composite for the whole hospital, including a few departments like pediatrics and Ob-Gyn that traditionally have a low occupancy rate.
- It is an average for the month, including high periods (Monday through Friday) and low periods (holidays and weekends).
- It includes beds in two-bed rooms that are not really usable because of patient-mix problems (smokers and nonsmokers, male and female, and so forth).

The total utilization figure is not too useful in planning, however. Although it has meaning as an economic indicator (because 82 percent occupancy can mean that you are operating in the black, whereas 65 percent means you are running in the red), the percentage does not tell very much about the hospital's problems.

To analyze and understand what is happening and to get at the problems, you must again turn to a matrix. The first run of data is the simplest, crudest, and possibly the most important. The data will tell you at a glance how each department is utilized. Set up the matrix like the one at the top of the next page.

Available Beds Utilized in One-Year Period

Department	Number of Beds Available	Percentage Utilized
Medicine	50	80
Surgery	50	90
Ob-Gyn	30	45
Psychiatry	20	65
Pediatrics	15	20

It will be apparent from the matrix that the medical and surgical departments probably have waiting lists. Another key point that will also be observable: there are probably too many beds assigned to some other departments.

Other insights to the workings of your hospital can be gained if you carry this matrix a step further by putting three years' data into this simple format, like this:

Available Beds Utilized in Three-Year Period

Department	Number of Beds Available	Percentage Utilized		
		Year 1	Year 2	Year 3
Medicine	50	76	78	80
Surgery	50	90	90	90
Ob-Gyn	30	75	60	45
Psychiatry	20	45	55	65
Pediatrics	15	20	20	20

You can see some interesting things going on:

- Medicine looks solid and is growing.
- Surgery is probably at the limit of its capacity. It needs examination; you may not be meeting the community's needs.
- Ob-Gyn is in a precipitous decline. You should find out why.

- Pediatrics utilization is low, and nothing is happening. Is the community trying to tell you to close it down, reduce the bed complement, or what?

The data above are simple to get and to put together. They tell you a lot about what is going on and, more important, they start to show you what questions you should ask.

Understanding Your
Medical Staff

Most of the questions raised by studying the hospital's utilization rate can be answered by studying the medical staff. You have discovered something important if you find your medical department draws 80 percent of its patients from the immediate community and 10 percent from each of the next two closest areas, but 50 percent of your surgical business comes from outside these areas.

You have discovered that you probably have on your staff a surgeon, or surgeons, who are drawing referrals from outside the normal trade area of your hospital. As a trustee, you should look carefully at this information, because you may have a strength on which to build a larger department than you now have. In addition, you have some risk. If the surgeon is a 63-year-old high-volume producer, you can anticipate a large drop-off in your business two years from now. You might want to encourage him, one way or another, to add some younger physicians to his practice.

The point is that you need to understand what is happening among your hospital's medical staff. Once you understand, but not before, you can begin to influence the future composition of the medical staff. This in turn enables you to build around your hospital's strengths and correct its weaknesses.

Now, make another matrix of the age distribution of your physicians, as shown on the following page.

This valuable and simple study involves a little ABC logic like this:

A. Doctors put patients in the hospital.
B. Older doctors eventually leave the staff, and, based on age, their departure is generally highly predictable.

C. If there is a high percentage of older doctors, it is relatively easy for trustees to forecast problems in the years ahead.

Age Distribution of Medical Staff, by Specialty

Medical Specialty	Number of Physicians					
	Total	Under 30	30-40	40-50	50-60	Over 60
Surgery						
Internal medicine						
Psychiatry						
Family practice						
Ob-Gyn						
Total						

A specific example is shown in the table below.

Age Distribution of Medical Staff, by Specialty

Medical Specialty	Number of Physicians					
	Total	Under 30	30-40	40-50	50-60	Over 60
Surgery	20	2	3	4	5	6
Internal medicine	15	1	2	3	4	5
Psychiatry	5	2	2	1	0	0
Family practice	10	3	1	1	1	4
Ob-Gyn	6	1	1	1	1	2
Total	56	9	9	10	11	17

What do these numbers say?

First, note that the figures indicate this hospital's medical staff is aging. Although there are many physicians in their prime, there are also a number who are about to retire.

Second, look at the psychiatrists; they are all young. Maybe a very healthy sign. Maybe a good group to build around.

Third, look at the family practice physicians. The figures show a bimodal distribution, that is, a distribution with two peaks. The distribution demonstrates why it is useful to work out this matrix. If you asked the chief of family practice, "What is the average age of your staff?" she would respond accurately, "42½." You would be lulled into complacency at a time when alarm bells should be ringing. The fact is that 40 percent of this important group will retire within the next couple of years.

In reality, you should make a much more detailed breakdown of specialties. For example, the surgical staff should be divided by subspecialty.

That is one attempt at understanding the medical staff composition. Here are other suggestions.

Where Our Doctors Live

Medical Specialty	Town A	Town B	Town C
1			
2			
3			

If the doctors on your staff must drive past three other hospitals to get to yours, that is a risk you want to know about.

Where Our Doctors' Offices Are

Medical Specialty	Our Medical Office Building	Another Hospital's Medical Office Building	Other Location
1			
2			
3			

Where Our Doctors Practice

Medical Specialty	Our Hospital	Tender Care Hospital	Loving Arms Hospital
1			
2			
3			

This information is often critical. If doctors work exclusively on your staff, your situation is much different from a hospital whose doctors split their time among several staffs. In such circumstances, your medical staff may have split loyalties.

Finally, a simple matrix gives information about trends in your hospital. It gives the name, the number of admissions for the current and previous two years, and, most important, the trend of admissions by each physician in your hospital.

Number of Admissions to Our Hospital, by Individual Physician

Name	1983	1984	1985
Physician 1			
Physician 2			
Physician 3			

The trend of admissions by each physician is what you should be really curious about. A doctor whose admissions have gone from 200 to 150 to 125 is telling you something. He is asking you to inquire "What's wrong?" and "What can we fix?" If you don't ask those questions, his admissions will be zero in a few years. So this is an important monitoring device for the long-range planning committee's examination of the medical staff.

Prospective Pricing and Medical Staff Relations

There is another way to look at and sort your physicians, and it is going to cause problems for the hospital, its board, and the physicians.

In the era of DRGs and prospective pricing—the code words used by the government agencies to describe the setting of pricing levels allowed for various treatments provided to Medicare patients in your hospital—you are going to have to look at your physicians in another way. Assume that you will be paid $1,000 for the treatment of a certain medical problem and that four physicians on your staff are authorized to manage (or treat) the problem. Each physician has handled twenty cases over the last six months, and in all cases the medical result was good. But under examination you discover that each of the doctors has used different tests, followed different procedures, ordered different drugs, and there has been some variation in the lengths of stay.

The hospital's accountants add it all up and here is the result:

P&L for Treatment XXX

	Dr. A	Dr. B	Dr. C	Dr. D
Income	1000	1000	1000	1000
Fixed costs	200	200	200	200
Doctor-controlled variable costs	700	800	900	1000
Profit/(Loss) per treatment	100	—	(100)	(200)

This kind of analysis of physician utilization is probably either already under way in your hospital or being talked about. And it is going to force the hospital administration and board into an involvement in medical care that no one is going to be comfortable with. The doctors don't want to be second-guessed, the board is going to have to insist on the hospital covering its costs, and the administration is going to be thrust smack into the midddle.

It seems inevitable that board members need to be placed on the hospital's utilization review committees. From personal experience as a member of a utilization committee, I know that the board members — surprisingly — can help. Although they can't and shouldn't pass out medical judgments, there are a couple of things they can do quite well:

- They can keep the physician and administrative staff from unproductive wrangling.
- They can ask simple questions, such as "Did the patients of both physicians have equal results?" (If so, then it is hard to argue for the higher-cost procedure.)
- They can express a lot of sympathy, hold a lot of hands, while insisting that for the hospital to survive it must keep expenses in line with the payments it will receive.

Now, this is a book about planning the hospital's survival, so we should return to that subject. Survival is probably going to mean not just more planning, it is going to mean more involvement in the issues of medical care. And more involvement in *quality* of care.

Being an effective trustee has just gotten harder.

The Medical Office Building: The Answer to Everything?

A lot of hospitals think they have doctor problems. A lot of trustees put it this way, "We need to recruit more doctors." This concern is almost universal among rural and small-town hospitals, and surprisingly, it is often stated by the trustees of many big-city hospitals whose staffs number in the hundreds.

Most boards of trustees eventually arrive at the cure-all answer: "Let's build a medical office building." The presumption is that the reason the hospital does not have enough of the right kind of doctors is that it does not have a medical office building close enough to the hospital to attract them. It is a fair guess that hundreds of millions of dollars have been spent on medical office buildings, on the premise that nothing turns a doctor on more than an office near the hospital. That premise can be challenged with the rhetorical question, "What do doctors want?"

Doctors want to:

- Be effective doctors, able to prevent and cure illness, and able to feel good about themselves.
- Make a lot of money, as most of us want to do.
- Live in the general environmental and ecological area that appeals to them.
- Be able to contribute to society.
- Work with good equipment such as the kind they were trained to use in medical school.
- Cut down commuting time between the hospital and the office, because it wastes revenue-producing time. Hence, the interest, perhaps, in an office near the hospital.

69

- Enjoy tax breaks. This often means it is better to own an office than rent one from the hospital.
- Ensure "coverage" for their patients in the hospital, so that they can relax on a free evening, knowing that, if an emergency arises with a patient, there is a physician on duty ready to deal with it.
- Work with specialists and associates with whom they can get good medical results.

The point is a simple one: doctors are motivated by a *long* list of things, not by one single item, such as a good office near the hospital. The problem of attracting physicians isn't simple. As a result of the high and naive hopes of boards of trustees, many medical office buildings have been built, only to sit half empty for a long time. The medical office building on the hospital's property may be the answer to your prayers, but it isn't the answer to every doctor's prayers. Before you build a medical office building, you should:

- Ask 10 hospitals that have built a medical office building how many years it took to reach a break-even point (you don't even have to be concerned with profits).
- Get input from the doctors in your hospital. After they have persuaded you that they are excited and serious about renting space in your medical office building, ask them to sign a legally binding letter of intent.

The medical office building may indeed turn out to be the answer to your prayers. It hasn't worked that way in many instances.

Green Eyeshade Time

Somewhere in your planning process you must get out your green eye-shade and be a steely-eyed accountant in order to come face to face with the economics of each hospital department. This is not as easy as it sounds and might appear impossible in some hospitals.

As a trustee concerned with planning the hospital's future at a time when cost is the A number 1 issue, you cannot escape digging deep. The questions to ask are these:

- How much do we make, or lose, per patient day on each service?
- How much do we make, or lose, per procedure?
- How much dollar volume is each of our physicians responsible for?
- How much do we make, or lose, on each patient?

There are more equally worthy questions, but these illustrate the idea. Yes, Virginia, this is a series of questions a granite-hearted bank loan officer might ask, and only a cost accountant could answer. And yes, the questions are 100 percent oriented to the economics of hospitals and totally ignore the idea that hospitals are primarily set up to save lives. But the questions must be asked.

You should know in advance that the data are tough to get at, and most hospital data, unfortunately, are not organized in a way that makes the answers easy to find. You may discover you can't get the answers without installing an entirely new information or cost system. This prior knowledge may save you and your administrator some fistfights and frustrations with the accounting department.

The difficulty of getting data doesn't excuse you from asking the questions and working on the answers. Knowledge of your hospital's costs and the economics of different departments and medical special-ties is essential to cost containment. Knowing which things make money and which lose it leads to far better decisions — about pricing, about equipment, and about buildings. It is inevitable, and essential, that you keep performing many services whether or not they carry their own weight financially. But winner or loser, you should know which is which.

Not All Problems
Have Solutions

After you have dealt with the nuts and bolts and dug out all the facts, it is time to feed the planning process with ideas that will lead to superior planning results.

First, you must hack away at the clutter of cliches and tribal legends that will make the job of organizing your planning committee harder and messier than it needs to be. Start with the all-time favorite cliches in planning circles:

- *If you can figure out the problem, then it is almost solved.* This is one of those tidy little statements that, like all cliches, isn't always—or even very often—true. If you figure out, for example, that all that separates your hospital from solvency is $1 million, you may have figured out the problem, but you still haven't figured out the solution. The point is obvious: whereas in hospital planning it is often difficult to figure out the problem, the solutions are almost always harder to come by.
- *All problems have solutions.* This isn't true, and you will avoid a lot of unnecessary and unproductive head-banging if you understand it. There are a lot of medical problems for which there is no known cure. There are also a great many problems in hospitals for which there is no known cure. Identify and solve the solvable problems. Identify, contain, and watch the unsolvable ones. Your answer to these may be to learn to live with them in reasonable comfort, not solve them.
- *There are always answers.* You must learn to live with ambiguity, because sometimes there are no answers. Your success will be

almost in direct proportion to your ability to handle the ambiguity that exists in hospitals. Persons who insist you get your costs down but want the hospital to have all the necessary equipment on hand when their family needs it typify the kind of ambiguity you must live with.

- *Someone else is to blame.* It's the government. It's the Blue Cross and the insurance companies. It's the doctors. It's society. It's the bureaucrats. It's the unions. It's the hospital next door. Hey folks, sometimes it is *you*, the board. *You're* the ones. *You're* to blame. *You're* the problem. *You're* the ones who have to change.

The theme is this: don't force conclusions from your planning process too fast, don't go for closure of problems prematurely, don't push so hard for solutions that you get the wrong answer. Many words have been written about how you dig for facts and how you set up the facts in tables or matrixes that will lead to insights about your hospital. The reasons are:

- Most of the problems that hospitals have are well known, because most of them have already occurred in other hospitals.
- Most of the answers already have been discovered and proven sound in a lot of other hospitals.

One of your key functions as a leader of a survivor hospital is to correctly match the problem and the solution. You are not required to be a great creative genius to discover new problems never before known to humanity, nor are you required to invent marvelously innovative solutions, but you must be able to identify the problems correctly in order to develop the right answers. There is only one sure way to do this, and that is to take your planning team into that jungle of facts, fiction, findings, conflicting opinions, and wild-eyed legend, and emerge from it competent to accurately assess what is going on. It takes work and a lot of it. You must suffer and endure the fact-finding process if you are to succeed. There is no painless way to success.

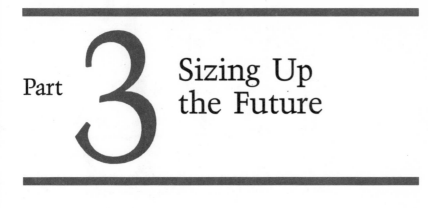

Part 3 Sizing Up
the Future

Doping Out the Future

Survival of your hospital is dependent on your ability to assess the future, to guess with reasonable accuracy what the needs will be in the community that your hospital serves and to anticipate a lot of other things, including what the government will do and what the big medical breakthroughs will be. You won't always be right, of course, but, if you really work at it, your chances of achieving a good batting average are excellent. This step in the planning process is easily the most interesting and may take the least time, yet it has great impact on the final outcome of your plan.

In the previous sections of this book, you learned to dig for facts about your community, customers, doctors, competitor hospitals, and a range of other topics. Now you must dig for the *trends* that will change those facts over the next 5 to 10 years. You must identify all the events or movements that will change and shape your hospital's future.

There is a simple premise that underlies this work. You do not need to be a genius to forecast the developments that will have an impact on your hospital in the next 5 to 10 years. You need only a good set of eyes and ears and a willingness to understand what you are seeing and hearing already.

Whatever will happen is already happening. This great truth should be chiseled into granite.

Trends in society start small and build gradually over a long span of years. They are not sudden at all; they just appear that way. You can figure out fairly well what the future holds just by being a good student of what is going on today. For example, a planning law was enacted in 1975. It was talked about, argued about, fought over in Congress for years. And this law had a string of predecessors. Now this law is moribund but has been replaced by more stringent regulations. And these, in turn, are very likely to be toughened again.

Viewed retrospectively, it is clear that the trend to ever-increasing regulation by the government of the quality and the cost of health care has been visible for 25 years. Your job is to identify the trends, figure out where they lead, and to predict how they will impinge on your part of the world of health care. As an example, the planning committee should try pursuing the trend of increasing regulation, extrapolating from the information it has to guess what future impact the trend will have on the hospital. Like this:

Trend: Increasing government control of the prices of hospital services.

Expected consequences in next 5 to 10 years:

- Consequence 1. Because the government is putting the lid on the income side, the hospital will be forced to control the amount and quality of services.
- Consequence 2. Controlling the amount and quality of services provided will set the hospitals on a collision course with their physicians, and new tensions will be created.
- Consequence 3. The government will pay an ever-increasing share of all bills incurred by patients. Government payments are generally slower than those of other third-party payers and require more handling. The hospital will therefore need more working capital.
- Consequence 4. The hospital will need to further enlarge its staff to respond to government requests for data and to process forms and papers.
- Consequence 5. More agencies of government will inspect the hospital.
- Consequence 6. A key management job will have to be established to coordinate all responses and activities that result from government inquiries.
- Consequence 7. Overhead or staff costs will probably go up faster than direct patient care costs, because of consequences 3, 4, 5, and 6.
- Consequence 8. Doctors will continue to yield ground to "planned medicine" and will steadily lose their cherished freedom.
- Consequence 9. Doctors' bills will be monitored, and some form of price control will become routine. Hospital rates are regulated now; the doctors' portion of health care costs will not be exempted for long.

- Consequence 10. Doctors' offices will be further affected by the rising tide of forms and data requests from the government. This will result in doctors forming into collectives or groups in order to be able to afford the management and clerical systems needed to cope.
- Consequence 11. The government will attempt to push some of the regulatory scorekeeping of doctors' incomes and practices onto hospitals. Hospitals and doctors will need to be careful not to get caught on opposite sides of the fence.
- Consequence 12. The health care system may develop into a *two-tier system*. One tier will be hospitals for patients who want to escape "the system" and for doctors who want to avoid the red tape of government. The other will be hospitals for everyone else. Your board will need to think about which way your hospital would lean, if such a split developed.

This list of consequences came tumbling out of one trend that was discussed in a single planning session and shows how just one group viewed the trend. But it is up to each hospital to decide for itself:

- What are the key trends?
- What kind of impact will they have on the hospital in the next 5 to 10 years?

Figuring Out the Trends

You should not leave the job of figuring out trends to government, your state hospital association, or outside groups. You have a better chance of being right about the trends that will have an impact on your hospital than they do. You can discover the trends if you:

- Read a story in the *Wall Street Journal* on a new piece of legislation and ask, "What does this mean to our hospital?"
- Listen to your liberal-leaning son who is home from college and bellyaching about "the system," and ask yourself, "What does this mean to our hospital?"
- Listen to a well-informed businesswoman as she blasts hospitals for the high cost of health care and ask, "What does that mean to our hospital?"
- Read headlines in the morning paper day after day and year after year and find that the politicians who are elected to office are the ones who promise "to do something about the high costs of medical care," and ask, "What does this mean to our hospital?"
- Listen to the President proclaiming that he will put a lid on the prices hospitals can charge customers and then read a forecast that costs in your hospital will rise 9 percent next year and ask, "What does this mean to our hospital?"
- Add these and 50 more messages together and ask, "What is society saying?" and "What do these messages mean to our hospital?"

You discover the key trends in society by listening and watching. Then you bring all these insights to your planning group, and together you try to figure out what the trends are.

Is it important to know? Well, is it important to know who will be paying your bills for the next 10 years? Is it important to know what the bill payer has in mind for you? Is it important to know what kind of behavior will be acceptable? Yes, it is. The survivors in the health care system 10 years hence have a very good idea of what society expects of them *now*.

Anticipating Medical Breakthroughs

Anticipating what's ahead makes most trustees throw up their hands, roll their eyeballs, and punt to the doctors. Unfortunately, this is where the doctors punt, too. But planning for medical breakthroughs is one of the easiest things you will cope with in the planning process. You already know most of what you are going to need to know.

Start with your own hospital's history. Find out what the important medical events were in the past 10 years. As a planner, you are interested only in knowing the breakthroughs that forced the hospital to:

- Construct additional expensive facilities or rearrange its available space
- Buy a lot of new, expensive equipment
- Hire a lot of people

In short, you should identify breakthroughs, such as building a new cardiac intensive care unit, buying a new scanner, or adding a new laminar airflow operating suite.

A typical 200-bed to 300-bed hospital might find that breakthroughs in medicine the past 10 years cost it:

- Two lumps of money in the $500,000 to $1,500,000 range
- Three lumps in the $50,000 to $500,000 range

Whatever you find in your history, plug it into your future. Add about eight percent per year for inflation. This is very much the way you do your household budgeting. You don't know which of your $500 appliances will need replacing next year, but you know you should expect one of them to poop out. You don't know if it will be the refrigerator or the washing machine, but you budget $500. This process will be familiar to most business people, because it is how they manage uncertainty. They expect to have some unknown expenses.

You should also find out what new techniques medical schools are using and what new equipment manufacturers are introducing, so that you will know well in advance what physicians will be seeking in the years ahead. There is a fairly predictable progression of technology. It starts in the medical schools; it spreads to the high-technology, highly specialized metropolitan clinics and hospitals; it moves on to metropolitan community hospitals; and last, it reaches hospitals in small cities and towns.

Figure out where you are in the progression, and then look upstream to see what is coming at you. An example might help. Twenty years ago, in many hospitals anesthesia was administered by nurse anesthetists under the supervision of a surgeon. Then medical schools began to train physicians who specialized in anesthesiology. As a result, young surgeons learned less about anesthesia and were trained to work in teams with the physician anesthesiologists. It wasn't long before that was the route most hospitals took. So look at how your newest physicians are being trained in order to know what is in store.

One further thought: urge the physicians on your planning committee to forecast the breakthroughs.

Considering Society's Changing Ethics

This book isn't the place to lecture about trustee ethics. That matter is between you and your conscience. The consideration of ethics here is strictly pragmatic, and there is no more pragmatic a fact of life to consider in the planning process than this: *Society's sense of what is acceptable behavior is changing rapidly.*

Society is moving rapidly, and the notion that it is now making the rules is an essential one to grasp. However, it is a notion that still has not registered with many trustees and doctors. It is up to the trustees charged with planning to discover what society's rules are and to bring their hospital in line with them. It is essential to the survival of their hospital. Take a look at the changing ethics:

- There is a considerable movement toward openness and away from secretiveness, from deals made in back rooms and from private business. There is a strong move toward operating in a fishbowl, where everything is on the record, out in the open, and conducted on the basis that, because your files may be searched, you might as well be out in the open with it all. This is happening not only in hospitals, of course, but also in government and many businesses.
- There is also a noticeable countertrend to openness and a wave of concern for privacy, such as the privacy of credit ratings and Internal Revenue Service tax returns. In the hospital, there are emerging concerns about who looks at medical records. Your hospital planning committee must assess this trend, always asking, "What does this tell us about the future?"

- There is a strong movement away from caveat emptor (buyer beware) and perhaps a move toward caveat vendor (seller beware). You doubt it? What do you think malpractice suits are all about? Malpractice problems are, in fact, a part of a much bigger trend. For instance, retailers, at least the bright, smart ones, now say, "We are the customer's purchasing agents." Retailers are no longer just pushing the merchandise that the manufacturers sell them but are taking it on their shoulders to quality-check the merchandise to be sure that it functions properly. They are taking it on their shoulders to send malfunctioning merchandise back to the manufacturer, putting their hundreds of millions of dollars of purchasing power on the side of the consumer, rather than the other way around. They are no longer simply selling merchandise to the customer with no further responsibility. "Seller beware" is becoming the new mode. The institutions that understand it will have a better chance of survival.
- There is a strong move away from hypocrisy, sham, dual standards. The public may be rejecting a double standard in health care, institutions, and government, saying that there have been two standards of health care, the kind that rich people got and the kind poor people got. Now, the public is saying that health care is a right and that everybody should get the same care. The behavior of manufacturers and the kind of statements they made in advertising 10 or 15 years ago were excused as "salesmanship," because exuberance and enthusiasm for one's own product were acceptable. Now the same kind of language will put the manufacturers in jail. Manufacturers, retailers, and others in business operate under stringent rules about what can be said and cannot be said in advertising. The double standard in this case has been eliminated.
- There is, simultaneously, a strong move *toward* a double standard in medical care. The government's efforts to control costs are causing many hospitals to resist subsidizing patients. Usually this means pushing patients who cannot afford medical care off to government-sponsored institutions. In effect the government is finding:
  —It cannot afford equal care for all.
  —It cannot bear to admit that out loud.

Those are just a few examples of the changing and confusing ethics of our times. A lot of people applaud the new morality. A lot of people also think it is much ado about nothing and regret the passing of the old ways. The point for you, as planners, is that you need to think about the environment you work in. Increasingly, a sense of what is acceptable behavior in today's and tomorrow's society is becoming good business for the hospital. On the other hand, a lack of understanding of what is acceptable behavior is becoming bad business. And if you are a planner who gets personal political preferences tangled up in the process or who feels obligated to resist the "new order," you are not going to help your hospital survive. You must be pragmatic and accept and understand reality — even if you don't like it.

The Muddle:
The Heart of Planning

Sooner or later in the process of putting your hospital's strategic plan together you are going to run into The Muddle. You will know you are there when:

- A couple of your committee members telephone you to say they think the whole project is a waste of time.
- Two of your most dignified trustees get into an embarrassing argument in the middle of a meeting.
- A previously uncommunicative and uncommitted physician suddenly starts crusading for a cause you thought had been killed off weeks ago.
- Your meetings are getting unruly and people interrupt or even holler. Decorum somehow has disappeared.
- The participants forget about projecting an image of importance and loosen their ties, take off their coats, and generally relax with each other.
- There is a general moroseness and a sinking feeling that the hospital is going down the tubes unless your little group does something about it.
- There is a general understanding that the big ideas that surfaced in the first few meetings were naive, even childlike.
- Most members of the committee are now attending every minute of every meeting, fascinated by what they are learning, scared to death that what they are learning is true, and beginning to doubt their learning will ever come to an end.

These are the classic signs of The Muddle. This is when your spirits will be lowest; it is also the point at which you are about to make a big breakthrough. When you see these signs, you can be confident the planning process is about to pay off. Here is what has been happening throughout the process:

- Each of the 8 or 10 members of the planning committee has brought a bright mind to the planning process.
- Each member has brought different disciplines and different viewpoints to the process.
- Each has been processing the data that have been dug out and the reactions of the other members of the group.
- Each has been through a process of discovering and examining the trends in relation to the facts about the hospital and has asked, "What do they mean?"

It is this mixing of good minds, different backgrounds, solid facts, and intelligent guesses about the future that leads to The Muddle — and it feels terrible. But interesting things are happening.

Recognizing When You Are Getting Red Hot

You will know you are hot on the trail, about to reach an important milestone or insight in The Muddle, when one of three things happens:

- Everyone in the meeting suddenly starts veering off, as though avoiding a big rock, or the conversation keeps bumping up against a big truth. Even though it is undefined and shrouded, you know it is there, because the subject of the discussion is constantly changed.
- A subject becomes too painful to discuss. Everybody knows the problem and may even know the solution, but it is too painful, too unthinkable, to voice.
- Everyone agrees too quickly that no decision can be reached without a lot more information or a research project being undertaken.

When these things happen, you should be wary and excited; you are close to something big. This is a magic moment, and you should get whatever is bugging the group out in the open. This is when you must press for a full discussion of the matter in hand, because strange things will come popping out.

As an example, a series of weekly breakfast meetings was set up for the trustees and the medical staff to discuss the pros and cons of bringing in full-time emergency department physicians to provide a higher level of medical care. At about the eighth meeting, a strange thing happened. The same arguments were continually recycled. The trustees kept pressing for additional full-time emergency department doctors. Although the physicians admitted that coverage was somewhat ragtag, they resisted fiercely. Their arguments ranged from the Hippocratic oath to the Communist conspiracy. The physicians made a lot of smoke and pyrotechnics, but finally the air cleared. What really had been in jeopardy, they believed, was income. They didn't want the emergency department physicians to swipe their patients. Once that fear had been articulated by a trustee, it took three minutes to find a solution.

It is this kind of simple clear insight that comes so hard but which is so important to the process of planning your hospital's survival.

Dealing with Sacred Cows

There are three subjects that ought to be on the agenda of every hospital's planning committee for a thorough airing once a year. They belong there precisely because they tie everyone up in knots and no one wants to talk about them:

- *Doctor economics.* The hospital may be causing problems for itself by scaring the daylights out of some physicians, as we have seen in the matter of hiring emergency department physicians. It may also be creating potential problems by overpaying a physician. In some states investigations are being cranked up to look at incomes of hospital-based physicians as a cause of skyrocketing costs. It is one subject no one wants to talk about. That is why it should be looked at.
- *Doctor feuds.* Conflict among factions of the medical staff is inevitable in every hospital with more than two physicians. The planning committee should assess the situation from time to time to see how much risk, if any, the hospital runs. If a couple of key physicians on your staff are about to toss in the towel because of a conflict of wills, your hospital is at risk, and you should know about it.
- *Religious overseers.* This is another untouchable subject for all hospitals sponsored by religious organizations. There is a real issue to be faced if religious leaders are dabbling where they shouldn't, or the denomination is annoyed and is about to pull out support because of a practice the hospital engages in. There may be an issue that the planning committee must discuss.

The planning effort is succeeding when issues like those can be brought into the open. There is an urgent message here. You are human, you are filled with love and compassion, you don't want to rile anyone, and you don't want to cause anyone pain. Your natural inclination is to withdraw and avoid painful discussions. You want to be a smoothie, a lady or a gentleman, a nice guy.

Folks, that isn't where the action is. Your objective is not peace and harmony, it is *not* to make friends or bandage wounds. Your objective is to figure out what is wrong, fix it, and then lay out a strategy for your hospital, so that in the future it can serve its customers effectively and efficiently.

When you smell a problem or an issue, drive right into the middle of it. Lay it wide open. That's what planning is all about.

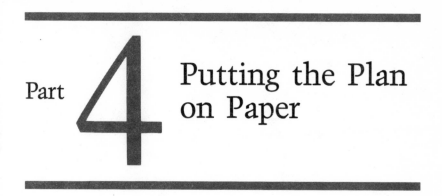

Part 4 Putting the Plan on Paper

The Mission Statement:
Where It All Begins

Planning is of little use to anyone until it is put into a tangible form. That means getting it down on paper. The place to start is the mission statement. The mission statement is easily the most important document your hospital will ever produce, because it establishes your direction, your tone, your size, your patient community, and your medical strengths. Yet 9 out of 10 hospital trustees, administrators, and doctors are unaware of whether a mission statement exists for their hospital, let alone what it says.

The mission statement should answer these questions and concerns:

- What does the hospital stand for?
- Where is it going?
- What can the hospital afford to do?
- What do patients expect of the hospital?
- What medical procedures is the hospital qualified to perform?
- Whom does the hospital serve?

The problem is that most hospital mission statements answer none of these questions. Instead they state, "The mission of this hospital shall be the provision of health care for all who enter . . . at the lowest cost." And that is the problem. If you sat the chairmen of 10 hospital boards of trustees at a round table and asked each to pass his mission statement to the person on his right, the chances are high that each mission statement would describe that person's hospital as well.

Most hospital mission statements are that general and that useless. They provide no direction, are so vague that they create no reactions, and are so general that no one would vote against them. Precisely for that reason mission statements have been the big yawner of hospital planning, but this cannot continue.

Hospitals have been remarkably sloppy in their statements of purpose. Such statements inevitably lead to drift and to wasted resources as the hospital tries to be too many things to too many people and jumps in response to each new political breeze or pressure.

A hospital of 50 beds cannot, and should not, attempt the same role as a 500-bed hospital, and its mission statement must reflect this. A small city hospital 100 miles from the next hospital has different responsibilities from one that serves the population of a major metropolitan area in concert with 25 other health care facilities. A hospital attached to a medical school has a role in society that is different from that of a suburban community hospital. The mission statements must reflect the differences.

Here, only slightly exaggerated, is the way the mission statement of a suburban community hospital often reads:

> The role of Loving Arms Hospital is to serve the needs of the sick who enter its doors seeking help, to provide that care in a compassionate way, and at a cost that is affordable.

The statement has the virtues of brevity and of keeping open future options by saying nothing and declaring no direction.

The mission statement that adequately describes your hospital's role will at the least deal with:

- The location of the hospital and the geographic area it intends to serve
- What medical specialty departments, which might serve as regional centers of treatment, the hospital has or will establish
- What the hospital intends to be or do in education
- The technological stage of medicine the hospital delivers
- How the hospital relates to other health care institutions, for example, independent of them, dependent on them, or a leader
- The hospital's religious preferences, if any (yes, they should be explicit)
- Cost, if the hospital has anything special to say
- Size—how big the hospital is or intends to become

Now, here is Loving Arms Hospital's statement of mission again, using this list as a guide.

> *Location.* Loving Arms Hospital is located on the corner of Main and Interstate Route 35. It is centrally located to serve as a community hospital for the residents of southern suburbs.

Level of care. It is an acute care, short-term general hospital of 250 beds, fully qualified to handle a broad range of medical, surgical, pediatric, obstetric, and gynecological problems.

Special strengths. The hospital has specialized strengths and is a regional center for the treatment of diabetes and renal diseases. It has a growing strength in emergency medicine.

Limitations. The hospital refers patients with long-term illnesses or psychiatric problems, or who need treatment for drug and alcohol abuse or rehabilitative medicine to other hospitals with whom we have working relationships.

Institutional relationships. The hospital provides medical and administrative leadership to the 36-bed Farmdale Nursing Home, the 112-bed Home for the Aged, the Pied Piper Drug Treatment Center, and the Center City Municipal Welfare Board. It also shares purchasing services with a group of 15 other hospitals.

Education. The hospital has clinical affiliations with the University Medical School and receives house staff from it. The hospital's teaching programs are designed to keep all clinical personnel at a proficiency level equal to other community hospitals of the same size. In addition, the hospital trains x-ray technicians and respiratory therapists.

Technology. It is the hospital's intention to be an early adapter of new equipment and technology after it has been proven necessary. This means not attempting to be first, but rather a quick second after the need has been proven for hospitals of this size and role.

Religion. The hospital is a nondenominational hospital whose background is Christian. It works with the chaplains of all faiths.

Cost. It is the hospital's goal to confine costs in ways that are not in conflict with good treatment. Its priority method for doing this is to attempt to provide excellent care for a broad range of illnesses whose treatment is within the scope of its skills, technological equipment, and resources. In addition, the hospital attempts to provide sophisticated skills and equipment in the narrow list of specialties already defined.

Now that is a mission statement. It tells people where the hospital stands on a lot of issues, what it is, and what it is not.

Organizing the Debate on the Mission Statement

The explicitness of the admission that your hospital is not the greatest, not the premier hospital, not the leader in all fields may have shocked you when you read the preceding section. You might want to "pretty up" the mission statement for external use, but it is important that at some point you talk in plain terms. You will find it tough going and hard to admit that any single part of the hospital will be anything but the most advanced.

To help you through an emotional and ego-bruising discussion, organize the debate by positioning your hospital between extremes. For instance, where does Loving Arms Hospital fit on these scales?

Medical Education

1	2	3	4	5	6	7	8	9	10

School
Nursing
Office

University
Medical
School

Ability to Treat Assorted Complex and Exotic Diseases

1	2	3	4	5	6	7	8	9	10

One-Man
Medical
Office

Mayo
Clinic

Starting with the list from the previous section, set up scales for a whole battery of issues. By doing this and making evaluations, the committee is obliged to decide what the hospital's position is. It can *not* get away with saying, "We're the best at everything."

Now refine this exercise. After you have declared where you are, go back and argue about where you should be. For instance:

Staff Education

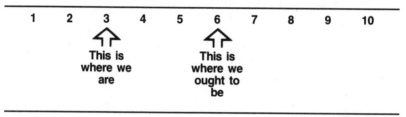

Another exercise that will also help you evaluate your hospital objectively is to position yourself in relation to other hospitals:

Emergency Medicine

1	2	3	4	5	6	7	8	9	10
⤊				⤊					⤊
Munificent Municipal (hangnails only)				Tender Care (middling abilities)					Loving Arms (the best)

Scaling your hospital's abilities and ambitions in this way will help you confine the emotionality of mission building and reach reasonably definitive statements.

If you can survive about three meetings on this subject, you have made a magnificent start—in fact, much more than a start, if you do the job really well—because your long-range plan is almost complete.

Everything else is easy. Although your mission statement should fill less than a page, it alone should set a course for years ahead. The mission statement is about 60 percent of your whole job of putting your plan on paper; the other 40 percent will then fall into place. In short, this part of the process is worth a lot of effort. Do it superbly, and the rest is easy.

Euthanasia in the Boardroom

Low occupancy in the hospital inevitably spawns new programs, many of which are introduced with the twin hopes that they will meet a real need in the community and improve the utilization rate. Innovation and a willingness to attempt new programs are essential to the survival of hospitals, because meeting community needs, filling beds so that costs are spread, and keeping room rates down are ever-present concerns. However, survival also demands that the results of new programs be monitored carefully and methodically.

In one instance, five new services were begun in a six-year period. Each was launched with a fanfare, a lot of hope, and much attention from the medical and administrative staffs. At the end of six years the score card read:

- One runaway success
- One marginally satisfactory program
- Three failures, as measured by community response and utilization, but all three services still open for business, propped up, and supported financially

Anyone experienced in the marketing of new products will tell you that one success out of five tries isn't too bad. That's the good news. The bad news is that three of those programs, although failing, had not been terminated at the end of six years. When programs fail, you must act decisively and purge the system. Failure demands euthanasia: survival demands that your hospital's mistakes be mercifully put to rest.

Whenever the board approves a new program, it accepts an obligation to monitor the results, at least annually. When the board perceives that a mistake has been made, it must correct the mistake. The rationale is:

- We went into this program with great hope.
- We gave it all we had medically and administratively.
- We sold it hard to the community it was intended to serve.
- It seems that the need we perceived was better served elsewhere.
- The time has come for the coup de grace.

Euthanasia, killing off mistakes, is an action seldom thought of, but it is essential to the hospital's survival. A big responsibility of the board is a willingness to say, "We tested the idea, and it didn't work." The failure of a program is not to be interpreted negatively; it is the natural consequence of trying new ideas in a tough environment, but you must correct errors. It is the only way you can have resources enough to expand to meet your real needs and go after the winners.

You exercise the responsibility to kill off failing programs by insisting that the sponsors of every new program accompany it by:

- *An assessment of the market:* "We have gathered data indicating that the community to be served wants the program."
- *A definition of success:* "We will consider this program to be a success when an average of 20 of the 24 beds set aside are in use."
- *A timetable of events:* "We expect to perform 5 procedures in the second month and 10 in the third month, and to level off at 15 to 20 by the end of the fifth month."
- *A projection of cash flow:* "We include a 36-month forecast of the positive and/or negative financial impact of the program month by month."
- *A definition of action courses:* "We will need to expand the program if it meets or exceeds expectations in six consecutive months. In this event, the board should be prepared to spend an additional $36,000. If the program does not operate at 50 percent of planned capacity by the sixth month, we must consider terminating the effort."

The principle is a simple one: survival of your hospital requires that you concentrate your resources on the facilities and programs that are most demanded by the community you have decided to serve, and that means getting out of failing efforts.

Another expression of this concept is to examine the whole hospital. Your driving concern should always be toward improvement, toward growth in quality, but all hospitals are not going to survive, and many shouldn't survive. By withholding approval for proposed projects, the state health planning agencies may squeeze some hospitals or hospital services out of business, so it might be more graceful and lead to a better result for the community if the board administered the final act. There are other advantages: for example, some acute care hospitals can probably be constructively converted for other levels of health care uses. It is better that the board find this direction now than face closing the hospital or a hospital service a few years hence.

Cost Containment

A book aimed at helping hospitals survive cannot escape addressing the subject of cost containment head on. It is what the fuss is all about. The world out there is speaking, sending hospitals multimedia, multisensory messages, and the word is GET YOUR COSTS UNDER CONTROL. The message is unmistakable.

So what is the problem? How come hospitals have been so unresponsive? How come they have been so insensitive to this message? The reasons are the corollary of the advice given by a child psychologist for the treatment of "spoiled" children. The psychologist says that parents should:

- Give consistent direction
- Be fair but firm
- Not threaten to punish, then not follow through
- Not give conflicting directions

But think about what has been happening:

- For 20 years or more society has been telling hospitals that their costs are too high but has gone right on paying the bills. That's *inconsistent direction.*
- Society has been telling hospitals that they must have the most advanced equipment because nothing is too good where health is concerned. Then society turns around and yells about increasing costs. That's *unfair attitude.*
- Society has made threatening gestures many times but failed to act. That's *lack of follow through.*
- Society has set up examples of ideal health care, such as the Mayo Clinic, the old family doctor, health maintenance organizations,

extended care centers, miracle-producing surgeons, and so forth. These models are in conflict. That's *conflicting direction.*

So although society has been making urgent noises to hospitals about costs, its statements have been overridden by conflicting signals. Like the spoiled child who receives conflicting direction, hospitals just went their own way. As with all spoiled children, you must look to the parents for correction. The problems are at least as much with society as with hospitals.

The message about cost containment has been heard for so long that it now lacks credibility. Administrators, boards of trustees, doctors, nurses, and others have been performing in an era in which increases in costs could be covered by increases in rates. The answer was to get the rates up, *not* get the costs down.

Through the President, the vice-president, Congress, 50 government bureaus, the state planning agencies, 100,000 bureaucrats, 50 labor unions, Ralph Nader, the news media, 1,000 consumer organizations, all sorts of business coalitions, and the health insurers, society is now saying, "This time we mean it. We won't let you raise your prices." It is a painful message, but it is there. Times have changed. Society does mean it. Hospitals must get costs under control.

The hospital board is probably in the best position to assume leadership in cutting costs. Those members of the board who are in general management positions in business or are owners and proprietors of their own businesses should be the nucleus of your costs containment leadership, because they have:

- Had experience with cost-cutting programs
- Heard the screams of anguish from middle management as personnel cuts were made
- Had to examine product lines for profitability and know how hard it is to cut the losers
- Heard the pained howls as cherished traditions were hacked away
- Heard the sales force rise up in protest to proclaim that the "competition will kill us if we cut back"

There are other subtle, but important, reasons to involve the board. Cost containment, that is, really effective control, will inevitably lead to reduction of programs and services, behind each of which are human beings who believe in them totally. Conflict is inevitable, and tough decisions are necessary.

Until now, hospitals have dealt mostly with the easy decisions. The first wave of cost cutting has involved purchasing practices and a lot of other items under the control of the hospital's administration. The next wave is going to involve bigger dollars and much bigger problems because it will mean invading the territory the doctors control.

The board must be the spearpoint, the bad guy, so that the administration can continue to operate effectively with the medical leadership.

Sensible, directed, and productive cost containment can be attained in three steps.

- The hospital must decide what its mission is, what needs it will serve, where it is going, and where it is *not* going.
- The hospital must have a five-year plan, a strategy, because it must know in precise terms where it is going before it can sensibly cut anything. Unessential programs cannot be separated and pruned back until the hospital knows which ones are essential, and don't let anyone tell you *all* the programs are essential.
- There must be a cost containment committee of the board. You will be inclined to give the function to the finance committee. Don't. Most finance committees are not staffed with the kind of talent you need. This job does not call for CPAs, vice-presidents of finance, or bankers, but needs instead general managers, business owners, proprietors, and division heads of business. It needs the people who are experienced in making the kind of decisions needed.

If your hospital is going to be numbered among the survivors in five years' time, getting control of costs is another step it will have to take, no matter how difficult that task will be, and it will be onerous. Society has made it clear that it does not intend to cover ever-increasing health care costs. Survivor hospitals will have responded to that message.

Becoming the Low-Cost Operator: The Plank That Belongs in Every Strategy

Strategic planning deals with the future, and as you look ahead these facts stand out in sharp focus:

- It is going to be a lot tougher to cover costs in the hospital by raising prices.
- It is going to be very hard to improve income through increased occupancy when that is the game every competitor is also playing.
- It is going to be difficult to even hold occupancy at current levels for many hospitals in the years just ahead because there are so many forces at work to reduce hospital stays.

In situations like this, hospital boards need to look back into the grand history of business. When they do, they will discover this is the precise time to trim down the organization, look hard at each cost center and each profit center, and simplify the enterprise's mission so it can be managed more effectively and with less overhead.

In a word—get your costs down.

Becoming a low-cost operator is an absolute necessity for *all* hospitals at this time.

That means, first of all, finding out what your hospital's costs are for every procedure, for every activity, and that usually turns out to be hard.

It also means finding out the costs experienced by other hospitals, and that may prove even harder. (If you are going to be the low-cost operator, you have to know your competitor's costs.) And finally, the *really* hard part—doing all of the things necessary to get costs ground down to the point where you can say with conviction: "This hospital is going to be a survivor because our break-even point has been lowered, we have stripped out the nonessential activities, we have reduced payroll, we have reduced the costs of doing business, and none of our competitors can beat us."

Each hospital will have to tackle this task in its own way. But the starting point will be planks, which are written into the strategy by the board and which might read like this:

- *Plank.* Lower the break-even occupancy rate of the hospital from 80 percent to 65 percent over the next five years. (Each hospital has to figure these rates out for itself, of course.)
- *Plank.* Become the lowest-cost operator in our trade area by systematically reducing the costs of running our hospital as measured by all indicators of productivity.
- *Plank.* Examine each activity in our hospital and make sure it is a "keeper" in our long-term strategy. If the activity or service does not fit the hospital's mission five years from now and it loses money besides, it should be high on our "hit" list.
- *Plank.* Examine all services and activities of the hospital and eliminate all those that threaten the future of the hospital because of high cost or that are unimportant to the treatment of patients.
- *Plank.* Examine all capital expenditures and give preference to investments that can be shown to reduce the cost of operation.

These are just examples, but they indicate approximate direction from the board as expressed by planks in the hospital's strategic plan.

It is this simple—the hospitals that fail to achieve lowered costs of doing business will not survive in the competition that is at their doorstep.

Appreciating Your Strengths and Looking Your Weaknesses in the Eye

Not all hospitals are created equal. Not all hospitals are great. Not all hospital departments are equal. Not all hospital facilities are the equal of their competitors', nor are the people who staff them.

This statement is intended as an antidote to the tendency to level out everything with generalities and as encouragement to you to explore and understand the differences in people, facilities, and locations you are concerned with at your hospital. These differences quickly divide into the things your hospital has going for it, that is, its strengths, and the hospital's shortcomings, its weaknesses.

You should know your hospital's strengths, because these are building blocks for the future, the assets you've got to work with. The weaknesses, of course, are on the negative side of the ledger. To discover them, you need to take two steps that are relatively painless but important to your final plan.

- Put your mission statement on a chart on the wall. Now get your planning group to list the hospital's strengths and its weaknesses. Without the mission statement in front of you, you can't tell the weaknesses and strengths apart. For instance, if your mission statement declares that the hospital's role is to specialize in mental health problems, the treatment of drug abuse, and the diseases of adolescents, the big program you have for the treatment of elderly patients in the neighborhood won't make it as a strength, even if it is medically and financially successful, because it neither fits the mission nor supports or enhances it. What you thought of as a strength is in reality one more thing to be corrected.

- Write everything down. Unless the strengths and weaknesses are explicitly articulated, every discussion and every argument will be recycled. Decide, then write down what the strengths and weaknesses are.

In the light of the work you have just done, you must be willing to change your mission statement. If the mission statement is in conflict with a major strength of the hospital, something has to give. Either the strength must be abandoned by declaring it to be no longer consistent with the hospital's role and objectives, or the role must be changed, but under no circumstances should the hospital try to live with the inconsistency.

Understanding your strengths is one key to survival. Looking your weaknesses in the eye is another.

Problems, Issues, and the Rule of Three

At some point the planning committee should develop a list of the problems your hospital faces and the issues that must be addressed if it is to survive and perform in the years ahead. The first step is to collect and identify the issues, and there may be 50 ways to do this. The procedure you develop should not be complex, and you shouldn't overwork this step, because of its redundancy in relation to the identification of the hospital's strengths and weaknesses discussed in the preceding section.

This step tackles the planning process from a different angle in an attempt to narrow the margin of error and increase the probability that what ails the institution has been correctly identified. The best procedure is for each committee member to work independently on the list of problems, beginning with the problems that exist and must be solved if the hospital is to progress. A second list of long-term problems that the hospital will face 5 or 10 years from now should also be made by each member. All the lists should then be sorted into two master lists: one for immediate problems, the other for long-term problems. The advantages of starting the process with individual efforts and ending it in a group are:

- A much longer list will be produced, and that in itself makes better odds that more problems will be aired.
- Certain problems will appear on many lists, and that will tell you something. Other problems will show up on only a few lists.
- Clusters of problems will emerge, and other patterns will appear, and these can provide useful information.

To illustrate the last point, suppose that on a list of 50 problems these 6 items appear:

- The hospital needs to attract more young, board-certified doctors of internal medicine.
- The hospital is in danger of losing its residency program in internal medicine.
- The director of medical education cannot get the cooperation he needs to maintain an effective teaching program.
- Doctors are angry because the cardiologist who reads all the cardiograms is slow, unavailable at night, and won't bring in another physician to his group.
- The cardiac intensive care unit is working at capacity and often has to accommodate patients in the hall. It is poorly designed.
- Turnover among nurses on the medical floors is higher than in other areas, and in the cardiac intensive care unit it is astronomical.

Remember those six problems are interspersed with a lot of other problems — everything from fire the board to fix the boiler. So you should build lists of clusters of like-sounding problems. By building a cluster, it becomes immediately apparent that all of these statements are really hitting the same problem from a different angle. The real problem (in this real-life case) was a crusty, irascible, tyrannical chief of internal medicine who intimidated the nursing staff, terrorized the administrator, scared off every potential young physician within a hundred miles, and did all the work in cardiology himself. The problem was how to control this physician.

That's the value of making the lists. They help the planners to get below the surface of the problems and into the substance.

Now, the Rule of Three.

The initial list of problems can easily have 100 entries. It is overwhelming. The list of clusters, or key problems, will almost certainly have 10 or 15 entries. At this point it pays to spend as much time as is necessary to rank this list by placing the most urgent problem at the top and the least urgent at the bottom. When you are satisfied that you have each of the problems in exactly the right order, draw a line under the third problem. This is the Rule of Three, and it states: Work on your top three problems. Solve them, and most of the others will go away.

Most organizations try to solve *all* their problems and wind up solving none. They spread themselves too thin and accomplish nothing. The Rule of Three is a device, a way to get your organization's efforts focused and cohesive.

The Plan

You have now been through the following series of steps:

- You have set up a long-range planning committee.
- You gave the committee a charge.
- The committee developed, studied, and absorbed many key facts about the hospital.
- The trends in medicine, hospitals, hospital communities, and society were investigated to assess the future of the hospital.
- A mission statement, which defines the hospital's role for the future, was argued through to a conclusion.
- Strengths and weaknesses were analyzed.
- Problems were identified and ranked according to priority.

The committee probably cycled and recycled through all of these steps. Planning is a learning process, a process in which learners are encouraged to let their perception of today's real world interact with their ideas about the future, the world that might be, or the world that will be. All the ideas now must be brought together and put on paper. Probably much of the planning has been committed to paper already, and the real problem is to get it all together.

Start with the outline proposed on page 34. That outline was intended primarily to provide a structure for the process of planning, not for the presentation of the final product, which is the planning group's thinking committed to paper. This outline should look like the one that begins on the following page.

Each hospital will tackle its plan a little differently, but the following plan will get you started.

Hospital Planning Document

Major Section	Key Topics	Comments
1. History and background	Key events since hospital founding Short summary of corporate ownership Description of present facilities Names of members of board of trustees Names of doctors on medical staff and their specialties Brief key facts about hospital	This is a short back-grounder. Write it for people learning about your hospital for the first time. Brevity is critical.
2. Planning perspective	Purpose of this plan Methodology used to prepare it Special research done Who did the work (members of planning committee) Who endorsed it	Be brief. This isn't the meat of the plan.
3. Mission	Old mission statement New (and much more explicit) mission statement	This section should also be brief, but these are the most important pages in the plan. Use exquisite care in language. Be aware this is the critical "sale" you must make to the board of trustees, the medical staff, and the community. Explain that the supporting data follow.

(continued)

Major Section	Key Topics	Comments
4. Place in community	Map of community showing location of all health care facilities, trade areas of each, including your hospital and bed counts	This section will be a long one. Show one table on each page and summarize the table in one paragraph on the same page.
	Detailed maps showing your hospital in relation to adjoining neighborhoods	
	Detailed maps showing your strong departments relative to other hospitals (by bed or procedure counts, and so forth)	
	Tables, as needed, of patient origin, utilization, referral physicians, and so forth	
5. Relationships with other health care institutions	Relationships you now have formalized with other institutions or agencies	This is an important section; be careful. Be sure to show how these relationships fit your mission.
	Relationships you plan for the future	
6. Strengths to build on/problems to solve	Depend on your hospital	This section will usually be an important one and will support your mission statement.
7. Goals/objectives for next 5 years	Depend on your hospital	Be brief.
8. Alternative planning solutions and final recommendations to achieve goals and objectives	Show three well-thought-out, plausible planning concepts you have looked at, explain consequences of each	Whether you show alternatives is optional. However, it is often helpful to explain some of the courses of action that were rejected.
	Final recommendation	
9. Mission	Restate the new mission	The mission statement is the single most important statement in the plan. End the document with a restatement of it.
10. Exhibits		This is where you stuff all the leftover tables, maps, and data developed during the planning process. In general, keep your plans thin and exhibits thick. Keep the main document tight.

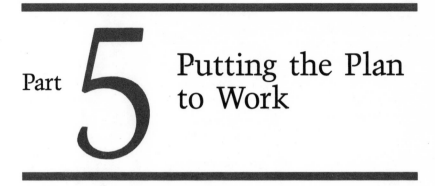

Part 5 Putting the Plan to Work

Selling the Plan to the Hospital

On page 31 it was stated that the 25 percent plan that gets 100 percent commitment is a winner, but the 100 percent plan that lacks commitment is a guaranteed loser. Now the word *sell* should be used. If you fail to sell the plan to all the doctors, trustees, nurses, managers, and employees of the hospital, your planning effort has been just fun and games—an interesting and stimulating intellectual exercise with no payoff. It is your obligation and responsibility to sell, or communicate, your plan and get the commitment of all those who must act in concert to make things happen.

The techniques that have been described in this book are designed to produce a solid plan and to generate commitment. Step by step, you should have gained understanding of and commitment to the hospital's objectives, because the planning has been done by respected leaders of the board, the staff, and the administration, all of whom have considered each side of every issue, aired the problems, reached conclusions, and made decisions.

In addition, you've had contact with people in the hospital, where there should be a fair awareness that planning is going on. Moreover, the rumors on the grapevine should have a high degree of accuracy, so there should not be any big surprises in the final recommendations. Thus, the climate should be good, and your final sale should not be difficult. That's the way things should be, and once in a while they really happen that way!

Your plan is the key to your hospital's future, so once the planning committee has the strategy, or plan, in hand, it must prepare a meticulous plan of communication. The power centers and the channels of communication are different in each hospital, but keep these things in mind:

- Don't bring the plan to a vote for adoption until the voters are ready. This means you must presell your plan, using one-on-one or small-group techniques, until all members of the board and hospital staffs have been reached.
- Be sure to have interim progress meetings with the board and hospital staffs while the planning is going on so that you can hear their comments, and they can later feel a sense of ongoing awareness.
- At the final big meetings of the board and the hospital staffs, be sure you have respected spokesmen, respected seconders, and the strongest leaders to do the selling. In most instances, these should be the ones who did the planning. That is why so much emphasis was put on getting those individuals involved and getting leaders who would be able to speak with authority and conviction.
- Show and demonstrate the depth of the work, but don't go into too much detail. Use expert visual techniques so that you can explain difficult concepts.

The purpose of this section is to emphasize the word *sell*. The reason is apparent. Your hospital, your community, and the patients who will use your hospital need that plan you have just produced, in place. The plan that isn't sold, isn't acted on, is for all practical purposes no plan at all, so selling the plan is a vital part of the planning process. It is the difference between oblivion and survival for a fair number of hospitals.

Saying It in Plain English

Saying it in plain English is the secret weapon of planners who play to win.*

Most hospital communication is laced with the acronyms, abbreviations, and jargon of the industry. It is further burdened with the language of planners, of new MBAs, and of the legal and accounting professions. Throw in a liberal sprinkling of medical school terminology and what you wind up with is some of the most pretentious and densest prose ever put down on paper. That's the language of the health care industry. It is some of the least communicative writing in America today. And it is a totally unnecessary hurdle to communication.

Make sure your plan is written in plain English. If you can accomplish that you will be able to reach the insiders better because most of them are baffled by the language too. But, most important, you will be able to communicate with all the people who are going to have to act on the plan:

- Board members
- Doctors
- Nurses
- Newspaper reporters
- Government personnel
- Employees all over the hospital
- Benefactors and potential benefactors
- Patients and their families
- Potential patients

---

*For more information on this topic, write to the Plain English Forum, 1185 Avenue of the Americas, New York, NY 10036.

If you start with the premise I do—that the plan that does not get acted on is a total waste of time—then communicating it is a top priority item on your planning agenda. That gets you straight to the art of writing in plain English, making sure your strategic plan is easily understandable.

This is not as simple or as easy as it sounds. In fact it is hard work at most hospitals, because the problem is not recognized by those who have learned to write and communicate with other insiders in hospitalese.

This recommendation is made to you: get a writer, a professional communicator to take the plan, organize it, translate it into plain-jane colloquial English. Zero jargon. No treasured hospital acronyms. Few words over three syllables. Short sentences. Short paragraphs. An understanding that brevity counts, and that usually people who try to communicate everything they know wind up communicating nothing.

Getting your plan translated into the language everyone can understand will take you a long way toward selling the plan, getting the action you are working toward.

Do it.

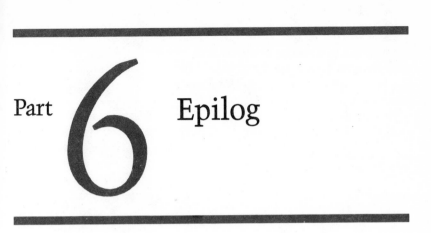

Part **6** Epilog

The Result of a Trustee's Work Is Patient Care

If inadequate patient care is being delivered in the hospital, there is no way for the board of trustees to claim that it has done its work well. There is no way to duck that responsibility, and it comes as a considerable shock to most trustees. Most trustees want to lay it off on the doctors or the nurses or the administration. On everybody but the trustees.

But if trustees start with the premise that the objective of the hospital is to cure the sick and help prevent disease, they very quickly come to the conclusion that they have something to do with health care. If you look at the legal responsibility of trustees, you very quickly find that the courts hold boards of trustees accountable and responsible; so, yes, trustees do indeed have a responsibility for health care.

This statement leads directly to this thought: your planning efforts should show up in improved care, care for more patients or more kinds of problems at lowered costs, or some combination of these possibilities. The obligation of the planning committee is to set up measures to ensure that performance standards are improved.

As part of that process, you must set patient care objectives for the hospital, and they should be measurable. There will be many measures to consider, and you should monitor your performance and, indeed, everything else, through the patients' eyes.

I am leaning hard on you to accept the responsibility for patient care not because it is your legal duty, but because ensuring that the hospital is competent is the principal moral and ethical obligation of trustees.

In the long list of expectations society has of its hospitals, nothing comes ahead of competence. Competence is an important measure of the hospital's performance and of its planning process.

Patients come to your hospital full of fear and full of hope. They are going to be denied some of their dignity and put in a position where they are unable to make good judgments on the basis of their own good common sense and knowledge. Suddenly they are dependent and defenseless. Under these circumstances they have the right to expect competence, the right to expect that you have provided properly for them, and the right to expect that people will do the right things at the right time. It is your ethical and moral duty to meet patients' expectations.

Your planning has paid off when patients talk about your hospital the same way you do. Your mission statement has become meaningful when patients can tell you on what occasions they would use your hospital and when they wouldn't—and their assessments match yours. Survival of your hospital is ensured when you and its patients think alike about its future.